Coping with Depression & Anxiety: Increasing Self Esteem

Overcome Depression, Sadness,
Get Your Confidence Back after
a Relationship Breakup and
Learn to Love Yourself Again
(2 Books in 1 Manuscript Bundle)

Stirling De Cruz-Coleridge

ISBN: 9781795772785

This declaration is deemed fair and valid by both the American Bar Association and the Committee of Publishers Association and is legally binding throughout the United States.

Furthermore, the transmission, duplication, or reproduction of any of the following work, including specific information will be considered an illegal act irrespective of if it is done electronically or in print. This extends to creating a secondary or tertiary copy of the work or a recorded copy and is only allowed with an express written consent from the Publisher. All additional rights reserved.

The information in the following pages is broadly considered to be a truthful and accurate account of facts, and as such any inattention, use or misuse of the information in question by the reader will render any resulting actions solely under their purview. There are no scenarios in which the publisher or the original author of this work can be in any fashion deemed liable for any hardship or damages that may befall them after undertaking information described herein.

Additionally, the information in the following pages is intended only for informational purposes and should thus be thought of as universal. As befitting its nature, it is presented without assurance regarding its prolonged validity or interim quality. Trademarks that are mentioned are

done without the written consent
and can in no way be considered an
endorsement from the trademark
holder.

TABLE OF CONTENTS

ABOUT THIS 2 in 1 BOOK MANUSCRIPT BUNDLE

Together these two books will help the reader to focus on the important things in life and how they can deal with what life throws at them, from a relationship breakup like a partnership, divorce or separation to losing a loved one, an illness or perhaps losing your job. These two value-packed books will give you the understanding and insight into how to deal with common problems and life issues, and how to enjoy life for the better and learn to love yourself again.

These books provide the reader with tools to handle anxieties and concerns whether it be for yourself, a loved one or special friend.

BOOK 1

GET BACK YOUR CONFIDENCE AND LEARN TO LOVE YOURSELF AFTER A RELATIONSHIP BREAKUP

(Self-Love,
Personal Transformation,
Self-Esteem,
Emotional Healing,
Self-Improvement &
Self-Confidence, Motivation)

Stirling De Cruz-Coleridge

This declaration is deemed fair and valid by both the American Bar Association and the Committee of Publishers Association and is legally binding throughout the United States.

Furthermore, the transmission, duplication, or reproduction of any of the following work, including specific information will be considered an illegal act irrespective of if it is done electronically or in print. This extends to creating a secondary or tertiary copy of the work or a recorded copy and is only allowed with an express written consent from the Publisher. All additional rights reserved.

The information in the following pages is broadly considered to be a truthful and accurate account of facts, and as such any inattention, use or misuse of the information in question by the reader will render any resulting actions solely under their purview. There are no scenarios in which the publisher or the original author of this work can be in any fashion deemed liable for any hardship or damages that may befall them after undertaking information described herein.

Additionally, the information in the following pages is intended only for informational purposes and should thus be thought of as universal. As befitting its nature, it is presented without assurance regarding its prolonged validity or interim quality. Trademarks that are mentioned are

done without the written consent
and can in no way be considered an
endorsement from the trademark
holder.

About This Book

This book covers the topic of how you can develop self-love and will teach you the different ways that it can transform you as a person.

At the completion of this book, you will have a good understanding of what it means to love yourself and be able to, hopefully, provide you with your need to live a fulfilling life.

Once again, thanks for purchasing this book, I hope you find it to be helpful!

Chapter 1 - Dealing With Pain

A divorce or any relationship breakup is one of the most emotional and stressful experiences that can happen in anyone's life. Whatever the reason for it is, it will always leave a scar in your heart. It might take a while, but moving on is possible. There are things that you can do to get over the stress, sadness, and pain that you felt because of it. Experts say that the first step to moving on is acceptance. You must accept the reality that you are no longer part of the other person's life, and you are hurting emotionally.

There are people who often say, "I'm okay" after a breakup even though they're still hurting inside. You shouldn't do this! Denying the reality of your situation won't help you move on. The pain in your heart will remain until you deal with it properly.

Why are breakups so painful?

Romantic relationships are composed of beautiful moments and memories. So, a loss of this kind of connection with someone in your life will greatly affect your being. In the span of your relationship, you spend a huge amount of time with him or her, so you're used to their presence. You'll surely miss them now that they're gone from your life. A lot of things become uncertain and unknown to you; responsibilities, routine, and your ties to the people closest to you and your partner.

Allow Yourself to Feel the Pain

You should know that it's okay to feel anger, confusion, resentment, and sadness. To fully accept the situation you are in, you must let your feelings out. Show it. If you want to cry, then cry your heart out-- do it. Let yourself grieve for the losses caused by the breakup. This is how you're going to let go of these feelings. You'll feel lighter after.

Resiliency

Resiliency is the capacity of a person to easily adjust to negative events in their life. It should help them balance his self, emotions, feelings, and decision. After the hardships, he should still manage to maintain functioning on both a physical and psychological level.

People who are resilient pay more attention to giving their inner self-strength. This is why they are prepared to face life's problems. On the other hand, people who are not resilient are easily swayed by difficult situations, overwhelmed by problems, and can't balance their physical and psychological health.

Having this trait does not necessarily mean that you won't face any difficulties, but it what it does is give you the fortitude to still find enjoyment and happiness after experiencing a divorce or breakup.

Resilience is not an inborn trait; you can develop it through experience. It all depends on how you handle the challenges that come your way. Here are a few steps on how you can develop resiliency in life:

1. *Be emotionally aware.*

The reason why people are overwhelmed by problems is because they do not know their inner self and the capacity of their feelings. As you grow up, you must slowly learn more about yourself, your personality, and characteristics. In that way, you will know how to react to life's challenges.

To do that, you can start by writing in your diary or journal. Write down the events of the day. You should note down how you behaved and handled every situation. Evaluate yourself and indicate whether you did the right thing or you just let those situations affect you negatively.

2. *Ask for supportive relationships.*

Any individual would need other people in his life. Some people may handle themselves very well, and they are independent, but it does not mean that they won't need support from the people close to them.

If you are experiencing a low point in your life, then you need your friends and family who can help lighten up the load. They will give you much-needed advice and encouragement to help you cope up with the stress. In this way, you will not feel that you are alone. There are still people who are willing to help you.

The emotionally healthy people know how to ask for help so they won't

carry the entire burden by
themselves.

3. *Be positive.*

Ensuring a positive attitude will get you through every obstacle. It is your way of encouraging and strengthening yourself. Though having social support is good, you still need positive strength coming from your inner being.

If challenges do come your way, you can easily yourself, "Stay strong!" or "I can do this!" These are just simple acts of courage, but if you believe them, then they will be of great help in overcoming the negative situations.

4. Know how to control yourself.

If you develop the ability to control your responses to different events in your life, then you will be more resilient to difficulties. While the positive and negative occurrences in life cannot be controlled, you should know how to react better. You always have a choice this in every aspect of your life.

Do not be swayed by the difficult circumstances. Instead, face and learn from them. It is your call if you will be weaker or stronger after every adversity.

5. Be optimistic.

It is about seeing things from the right perspective. People will experience both sadness and happiness, but the optimistic ones are the people who know how to maximise the positive and minimise the negative things in life.

6. Do not give up.

If you are in a difficult situation, you will overcome it. You need to know how to do it. But the most important thing is not to give up because you always have a way of defeating the obstacles. Just look around and see the people who are willing to help you.

Loving yourself is the first step to happiness. Without it, you can end up forgetting the value of taking care of yourself before anyone else. Invest in it by feeding your mind, body, and soul. You will be happy in doing so.

Here are a few tips and things you can do give yourself some much-deserved love:

- *Listen to your feelings.*

- *Have compassion for yourself.*

- *Be open to changes about what your self tells you.*

- *Surround yourself with loving people.*

- *Be kind to yourself and others.*

- *Manage your time and money wisely.*

- *Take care of your body and health.*

- *Look for a job that you love.*

- *Lead a balanced life.*

Chapter 2 - Emotional Healing

When talking about health, most people would think of physical fitness, rest and sleep. Others would think of nutrition and diet. These are all related to health, but only in the physical aspect. Fact is, most people are not aware that the mental and emotional state are also important parts of the overall well-being of a person.

Mental and emotional health are different parts of who you are as a person. Most people think that they are the same, but here are the things that separate one from the other.

Mental Health

It requires cognitive thinking which includes critical skills such as long-term memory, processing speed, logic and reasoning, visual and auditory processing, and the ability to keep attention on specific tasks.

The brain is primarily involved because it processes every bit of information that comes from the five senses. It takes care of how the body reacts and responds to external stimuli. Making decisions and formulating opinions are also part of mental health.

Emotional Health

It is defined as your capacity to understand yourself and how sensitive you are to your psychological experiences. This also involves how you control your feelings and emotions, including dealing with and influencing other people. This includes how you're able to bounce back from the difficult situations in life.

Every person would have a different response to emotional experiences. Younger people have less understanding of life, so they are usually overwhelmed by strong emotions. While the older ones are more able to control their feelings, they know how to handle difficulties better.

So, how do they differ from each other? Mental health helps a person process the information given by the brain for them to think and make the right decisions. Emotional health refers to the ability of a person to express his feelings and emotions appropriately. Though they have different functions in maintaining your well-being, they cannot be separated from each other. People often call them as the mind (mental health) and the heart (emotional health). They need to be balanced so you that you develop the right outlook in life.

When facing problems, you need to analyse the situation first. Ask yourself, "Why did it happen?" or "What are the mistakes I did?" After that, you can use your heart to make the right responses to the problem. That is how they work together.

Mental and emotional health needs to be taken care as much as your physical health. If you ignore them, you can end up experiencing psychological illnesses like depression, anxiety, worry, trauma, and even stress. If you're not able to process the information or control your feelings, it can end up cluttering your head. This, alone, is very stressful and can lead to more serious problems. And it can affect a huge part of your life, making it more difficult for you to move on from the heartache.

Having a healthy mental and emotional state does not always

guarantee happiness, however. Every person would encounter setbacks and adversities like disappointments and breakups as they go through life. They are inevitable. The only weapon you have is your inner strength. Happiness comes from your ability to listen to your own emotions and feelings and making the right responses to it.

How will you know if you are mentally and emotionally healthy?

Emotional health can also refer to your knowledge about your feelings and behaviour. So if you are aware of the things going on within you and can handle things more logically, then you can say that you are psychologically healthy.

Here are other factors to help you identify if you are mentally and emotionally healthy:

1. You are aware of your feelings and thoughts.

2. You are happy with the life you have.

3. You are content with what you have.

4. You have a positive attitude.

5. You have high self-esteem and self-confidence.

6. You are always prepared to learn new things and flexible to changes.

7. You know how to balance your work, relationships, and yourself.

8. You have set a purpose for yourself in this life.

9. You know your priorities.

10. You know how to accept mistakes and learn from them.

11. You know how to seek social support.

12. You can handle problems and get back up.

These are just some of them. You can ask yourself if these are present in your life and if they aren't? Don't worry! These are things you can always work on. At least now, you know which ones to improve and develop more when it comes to your own emotions and feelings.

Be Open to Supportive Relationships

Most of the strategies and tips stated above are done by yourself. But, to achieve the best emotional condition, you would still need others to accompany you on your "moving on" stage. People are not made to survive and live alone on this planet. They are meant to connect and relate to others and develop companionship.

Having someone who will listen to your struggles and suffering may help reduce the burden you are carrying. It is a way of releasing the heavy feelings and emotions that you keep bottled up.

It is not enough to just find a friend; you must look for someone who can also become your supporter and adviser. They must be willing to understand your situation and listen to everything you'll say.

Friendship is a give and takes relationship. If your friend is always there for you, then you must do the same for them. Remember that these people will eventually experience setbacks in life too so make sure that when the time comes, you're just as ready to listen and to be present.

The question is, "How are you going to connect with other people?" Here are some tips and strategies to consider:

1. Socialise outside the Social Media.

It is true that you can make friends through the social media, but it is not effective as meeting the person face-to-face. Personal interaction includes the emotions, tone of voice, facial expressions and gestures. Relationships in the real world tend to be more successful.

2. Go out and meet new people.

It is not good for your mental, emotional and even physical health to just stay at home all the time. You need to interact and widen your network to gain more friends and knowledge about your environment. Cherry-pick to surround yourself with people who are positive, cheerful, and engaging. You need those kinds of people in your life.

3. Join clubs, organisations, and other social groups.

This will help you turn your acquaintances into friends. These social groups are your bridges to different types of people. Think of this as your chance to learn from them and also share what you have. You can create stronger relationships with your fellow members, and it is a great opportunity to meet people with the same interests as you.

Take time to help others.

Helping other people gives a sense of purpose in your life. Being more fortunate than other people is already a great blessing. There are lots of people in this world who do not live a blessed life so you should have the heart to share your blessings with them. You can help, not only regarding donations and money but also through volunteering to different organisations that cater to them.

Moving On Emotionally

Be Kind to Yourself

The way you see and treat yourself will set a standard on how others would approach you. If you say bad things about yourself, it wouldn't be hard for other people to do the same. Remember that *"No one can make you feel inferior without your consent,"* says Eleanor Roosevelt. Therefore, love yourself, and then you can expect the people around you to be kind to you.

Learn to Forgive

Do not let the hate that you have for other people stay inside you. It can hinder your ability to love other people. Forgiveness is not about forgetting the bad things they did to you, but it is about letting go of the hatred and pain you experienced. It doesn't erase the past, but it will help heal the wounds it created in yourself.

Learn from the Good and Bad Situations you Experienced

Every circumstance you encounter in your life is meant to teach you something. There will be good and bad times, but both of them can make you a better person. So, whatever happens to you, try to discern what it taught you. In that way, you will be a better person. And when a bigger challenge comes your way, you will be able to handle it better.

Stop Caring About What Other People Say about You

They may say things about that are not appropriate for you. Negative things that can make you feel bad about who you are. Remember, if you know yourself and your truth, then whatever they say no longer matters. As long as you're confident, there's no need to worry about other people's opinion of you.

There will also be times when people would try to control your life. Stop thinking about them because you're the only one who knows exactly what would be the best option for you is.

Learn to Let Go of the Past

The things, people, good and bad experiences in the past are already done. You already learned what you could from them, so what you have to do now is to move forward. Do not let the past affect your present and future negatively.

Do not Fear Failures

Everyone is afraid of something. You may have a fear of failure or changes that may happen in your life. But the thing is, failing at some point in your life is normal. You wouldn't always succeed in the things you do. But, let it be a lesson for you, something you can use for your next task. The worst thing that failure and changes can affect you with is the fear of making another mistake. Never stop trying. A lot of successful people have failed a thousand times, but these didn't stop them from trying again.

Let Go of Regrets

"You only live once, but if you do it right, once is enough," said Mae West. There are things that you can't control in this life, so you must live your life the way you want it to. Give your best in everything you do. Learn from every mistake and failure. Never let other people control you. Just live your life to the fullest. And if you know that you did that, you can easily let go of your regrets.

Be Open to Changes

Change is the only thing constant in this world. Do not be content in staying within your comfort zone. There is so much more to learn and experience outside of it. Do not be afraid of the things you don't know because that is when you can learn and grow.

<u>Enjoy the Simple Pleasures of Life</u>

All the best things in this life are free. So, you don't have to worry about having not enough money because happiness depends on how you feel inside and not by the things you own. Learn to appreciate the small things that you have because they are the ones that can give you true pleasure in this life.

Chapter 3 - Letting Go

Do Not Cling to the Past

Ajahn Chah, an influential teacher of buddhadhamma, once said, *"If you let go a lot, you will have a little happiness. If you let go more, you will have a lot of happiness. And if you let go completely, you will be totally happy."*

Your "past" is already a part of your life. During that time, you may have experienced hardships, failures, criticisms, and many more. It is okay to look back at those moments of your life and learn from it. But it is not healthy to stay there, regretting what could have been. Learn to put the past behind you. Do not let it ruin your present and future decisions and goals. If you keep on lingering in the past, you cannot move forward.

Focus on the present moment and plan for the future. One that highlights YOU and not anyone else. It is important that you start doing things for yourself instead of depending on someone else's idea of what's good for you.

Sometimes, you might feel that something is missing in your life. Have you asked yourself what it is? If not, ask yourself about the thing what makes you motivated to wake up in the morning and go about your daily tasks. Many people only exist, but they are not living. Your purpose in life is what keeps you going; it's what helps you achieve happiness and success. It pushes you in the right direction where you want to go in the future.

Coming from a bad breakup might take away your sense of purpose. So to help you get back in the right direction, follow these steps:

Know Yourself First

Before knowing your purpose in life, you have to know who you are: your personality, traits, likes, dislikes, dreams, and passions. In this way, you will have a clear picture of what you want to become in the future.

You can even get a journal where you can write about your thoughts and perspective about certain things. When you read it, you will gain a better understanding of yourself.

List Down Everything You Want to Achieve

This is not only about material things, but also having a family or a good career. Write down the things that you love to do the most; your dreams, interests and passion in life. These are the things that you enjoy doing the most and the things that make you happy, even if you are not paid for them.

Contribute to the Society

Always try and look beyond yourself because you are here to contribute what you can to the society. Determine the problems and needs of the community you are in and find out how you can offer a solution. Lend a helping hand to someone when needed and work together with other people. Your interests and passions can make a difference to the people around you if used in the right way.

For example, you want to be a chef or restaurant manager someday. When the time comes, you can give back to the community by providing employment. You can hire people as waiters or cashiers in your restaurant. In your small way, you can help make a difference.

1. Look for Inspiration

There will always be people who have experienced the heartbreak you are feeling right now. These people have passed through their obstacles and hurdles before reaching where they are now. You can learn from their experience by asking for advice or help. If they are not within your reach, like world-known leaders or historical figures, read about their lives. There will always be material for you to absorb and take inspiration from.

2. Do Not Stay in Your Comfort Zone

Try to go out and see a bigger view of the world. There's so much to it that you might be missing out on because you are satisfied with staying at home. Explore the world! This way, you would be able to meet more people and experience things that can change you for the better. It is life's way of making you stronger and more confident in facing your fears. Take risks and know what you are capable of doing.

As you live outside your comfort zone, think of a better purpose for your life — something that will help not only yourself and your family but also other people.

2. Determine Your Purpose

Now that you have examined and evaluated yourself, it is time to figure out your purpose. It might change in the future, but what's important is that you are slowly picking yourself up and setting goals that depend only on you. This should help you regain power that you may have lost due to heartbreak.

Chapter 4 - Rebuilding Yourself

Self-esteem is about having faith in yourself; having confidence in your strengths and being honest with your weaknesses. It is also about self-respect because you show love and value to the person that you are. Self-acceptance is a major part when it comes to gaining self-esteem. This is because you have to know and develop your personality, attitude, and principles in life. Accept everything that you might discover about yourself; including the good ones and the bad ones because these are the things that make up your whole being. If you don't, you will end up facing failures and disappointments later on because of you either have low or high expectations about yourself. You will always strive for more, despite limitations, and that kind of attitude will get you nowhere.

For you to have a clearer understanding of self-esteem here is an example:

There are people who love cooking and want to be a chef someday. Since it is important to them, they will find ways when it comes to honing their skills and finding the information you need about cooking. They will also invest money in buying what they require to create the perfect recipe. When they set their minds on things that they value, they will do what it takes to achieve it. This trust in their abilities is what self-esteem is. You know what you're capable of so you push forward with what you want.

Your self-esteem will influence your purpose and decisions in life. It will motivate you to be the person you want to be in the future. It will also give you a sense of responsibility to better take care of yourself and health to reach your full potential. On the contrary, people who have low self-esteem are more prone to experiencing stress and depression. They feel hopeless and worthless because they do not know how to adjust and bounce back from life's problems.

Now that you have some understanding of what self-esteem is, and effect in your life, it is time to apply it in the right way. There are unexpected moments in your life wherein you need to make immediate yet confident decisions. Here are tips and strategies on how you can do that without second-guessing yourself:

1. Avoid self-doubt and believe in yourself.

Self-esteem is about valuing your talents, skills, and personality. So, if you don't have faith in yourself, then you won't be as assertive when facing the difficult situations in your life.

If you keep on delaying the process of reaching your goals, you will end up thinking of more reasons to not do it. You will lose inspiration and motivation because of overthinking things.

2. Challenge negative thoughts

Stop thinking about being helpless or worthless because this is just another way of telling yourself that you are not good enough. It degrades your self-esteem because you start to think that you don't deserve success or prosperity in life. Your negative thoughts will continue to affect your goals and ambitions in life if you don't do something about it.

Convince yourself that those negative thoughts are not true. Focus on your strengths because this gives you the confidence to do things beyond your expectation. You can even ask your family and friends to reinforce what you believe yourself to be; if they see positives in you that you have failed to pinpoint for yourself, then that gives you a much-needed confidence boost.

3. Give yourself credit for a job done well

Achieving self-esteem is a process. If you think that you have overcome a particular hurdle in your life, treat yourself as a reward for it. Use this as a way of reminding yourself that difficulties will eventually end if you work hard enough for it—the best bit? There's always something good waiting for you at the finish line.

Entertain more positive thoughts so you won't feel down about yourself. Spend some time reflecting and evaluating the events that happened during the day and highlight the good ones. It will help you realise that there are still good things to come and look forward to.

4. be open to good comments and praise about you

There are things that people notice about you which you might not even be aware of. Take some time to listen to them, especially the positive remarks that they give. It will help you gain more faith in yourself and the things you can do.

Simple and Fast Ways to Improve Your Self-Esteem

Self-esteem is not easily achieved because it takes a lot of effort and courage to face unfamiliar situations. You also need to work on your behaviour, insecurities, fears, and changes every day to see improvements in yourself. Reading a lot of articles and blogs about gaining self-esteem will not help you obtain it; you also need to take action.

1. Have a mantra

You can do this outside of meditation. Many people use mantras when you faced a difficult situation. You may have done this before unconsciously. Have you given yourself a pep talk before a big event? A presentation that's important to your career? There are those phrases that give you strength and confidence to face the challenges in front of you. It's always best to choose your own personal mantra, but some examples you can also use are: "I can do it!' or "I have prepared and practised for this, so there's no way I'm going to fail." Remember to say the words aloud or in front of a mirror. This might make you look silly, but it actually helps.

2. Talk to people close to you

Self-esteem can also be achieved through the help of others, especially those who are close to you. They know who you are, your strengths and weaknesses, so you can trust them to give you honest compliments and comments. They can also provide encouragement which should ease any tension and worry you might be harbouring.

3. Smile

Do it even when you don't feel like it. Then slowly, it will lift your mood. Frowning and having an emotionless face can actually end up worsening the tension in your body.

What is Confidence?

How do you differentiate confident people from the ones who are not? It's easy to spot them. Confident people are those who are capable of giving straight and honest opinions during a meeting. They are also among those who volunteer for difficult tasks like giving a speech in front of a large crowd. While these things might come off as pompous to some, if done with proper intent, they are a result of a positive attitude and mindset. Remember that being confident is not about bossing people around or showing off your intelligence and talent to other people.

Confidence is being brave enough to take action. One that does not give off a negative image, but inspires other people to have the same assertiveness in certain situations. People have fears, and it is inevitable. They all want to achieve success, but they do not have enough courage to reach for it. To be confident, you must act on these goals and dreams, without allowing the fears stop you from achieving them.

The more you gain the courage to do things, the more your confidence grows. It is a process that you can learn and build for yourself. Confident people can go further and achieve more success because fears along the way do not block them. It is about turning the positive thoughts into action. But do beware of arrogance, you might think of it as confidence, but it is not.

Self-Awareness

The first step in gaining confidence is at peace with yourself. You must know who you are and accept it. Discover your strengths and weaknesses, so you know what to improve in yourself. This way, you will not be sorry or have regrets if you fail or make mistakes on your way to healing yourself. People can make decisions that aren't good for them, it can put them in unhealthy situations, but this doesn't mean that you no longer deserve anything good. In fact, now is the time to pamper yourself even more. LOVE everything about you, flaws included.

Positive and radiant energy will continue to overflow from you because you are content and satisfied with who you are. Confidence will follow as long as you are aware of your actions. Know your goals and dreams so you can take even the smallest steps to achieve it without being afraid of the upcoming obstacles and challenges.

Practice Confidence

Self-confidence can be learned, and it is also attainable even by introverts and shy people. You just have to stay motivated and determined enough in practising it as part of your everyday life. Building confidence will lead you to success, and you can claim that it is your achievement.

Here are some steps to consider when it comes to practising confidence:

Everyone strives for confidence.

There are people who seem not to have any problem talking to people or performing on stage. But, if you ask them what they feel, they will tell you that they still get nervous and anxious when facing social situations. They are also struggling to gain confidence in every task that they do. These people are simply good at pushing all of those fears aside and taking the leap.

Focus on your strengths and weaknesses and do not compare yourself to others. They have their battles to fight which you might not even be aware of. Just strive to be the best version of the person you want to be; in doing so, you will gain happiness. Compete with yourself and get better with every challenge.

Identify your strengths, talents, and skills.

The reason why most people have low self-esteem is that they keep on thinking about the things that they can't do. After a toxic relationship, it is very easy to feel as if there's nothing positive about you. That you cannot do anything right—after all, you have been manipulated to think and feel this way. Move past that by focusing on your skills and talents. Write them down and determine your best abilities. Next, gain more knowledge about these skills. The more you improve, the more confidence you'll gain.

Gaining confidence is a process.

When you were still in school, you might have developed confidence through class reports, speech contests, and daily recitations. But, as you grew older, you realised that there are more challenges that would bring your confidence down. Relationships, for one, can greatly influence how we feel about ourselves. The wrong one can make you feel like you are not good enough.

This is not a dead-end. You must see confidence as a process. As you go through life, anticipate more social situations that will test your inner strength. Prepare yourself for what's to come so you will be ready and confident in facing it.

Help other people.

Another way of boosting your self-confidence is by making other people feel confident about themselves. Help make them feel better too through your compliments. You'll find that doing so actually makes you feel good about yourself as well. Giving and sharing positive vibes will help you build strong relationships with other people. Healthier ones that only work to push you forward.

Avoid people who bring you down.

Do not surround yourself with people who can't appreciate your talents and efforts. They will only negatively influence your confidence if you keep hearing their ill-intended comments and wrong judgments about you. If possible, remove them from your life because you deserve better. Give toxicity no room in your life. Instead, choose someone who will continuously encourage and support you even in during ups and downs.

Surrounding yourself with positive people will help you grow better as a person, and you can do the same with them too.

Do not be afraid to take risks.

People experience failures now and then. This is great as it helps them develop better strength and courage when it comes to the challenges they may face in life. It is inevitable and cannot be avoided, so what you need to do is gather your courage and learn how to get back up from the losses.

If you want to improve a certain area of your life, you have to go through the process. Sometimes, it will be hard and painful, but remember that these experiences are never without lessons. You will become a better person through them, just have faith in yourself.

*Expect the good things and think
positively.*

When you think of failure even
before the race starts, then you've
already lost the game. Expect success
in every situation you face. Always
believe that whatever happens, you
will get through it. You just have to
give you one hundred percent to
achieve what you wished for.

Have more faith and confidence to
reach your goals in life. Never allow
what has happened to you in the past
hinder you from this. Start doing
things for yourself instead of
depending on someone else to make
the decisions for you—think of it this
way; you are now responsible for
yourself. So make the most of it.

Chapter 5 – Personal Transformation

Another part of the process of moving on is Personal Transformation. If you just came from a bad breakup, there's a good chance that you'll feel ugly and unworthy. This can be a depressing state of mind and because of that; you might even forget how to take care of yourself. This applies to both your mental and physical state; both things which are important to your ability to move past the bad things and become a better person. So, while you're still working on your mental well-being, you can also do things to boost your physical confidence.

Treat yourself better, this is what most people would tell you and that's because there's plenty of truth in it. Haven't you heard? The best kind of payback is to start being a better version of yourself. Here are some tips that you can follow:

Start Eating Healthier and Choosing Better Food for Your Body

It is true that breakfast is the most important meal of the day. It gives you enough energy and strength to help get you through your daily tasks. It also helps the mind properly process all the activities you have for the whole day. However, some people skip breakfast because they think that it is just a waste of time to cook in the morning or they simply don't have enough time for it. It also makes them late for appointments and other schedules. However, doing so can lead to some pretty serious issues.

Some illnesses develop if you don't take your breakfast regularly. It can heighten your risk for diabetes and even heart disease. It also might also cause an increase in the levels of bad cholesterol in your body. Skipping breakfast can make you feel weak and tired for the whole day too. Did you know that this can make you feel much more stressed and irritable? It can make you feel worse about yourself too! Remember, everything is connected. If something affects you physically, chances are, it would also affect your mentality.

If you're dieting as part of your transformation, skipping breakfast is also a bad idea. Why? This is because it can also push you to eat more during the day. Can it easily cause you to snack more and the worst bit? If you're in a hurry, you have more of a tendency to reach for snacks that might be bad for your health. Fast-food, sweets and junk food are the most common snacks that people reach for throughout the day. Yes, they taste good, and you feel satisfied for a while, but it does not benefit you in any way.

All of that just because you chose to skip breakfast!

Now, do remember that it is not only necessary to have breakfast at the proper time. You should also make sure that what you're having is a healthy and well-balanced meal. You're not just going for energy here—you also need the important nutrients to help your brain function better. Did you know that choosing the right food can also make you feel happier? Certain food items stimulate the body to release what's known as 'happy hormones' which can make you feel brighter and more energetic — providing you with more clarity and the ability to boost transformation. So if you're going to eat breakfast, always make sure that you are getting all of the essential vitamins and nutrients that your body needs. Help your body, and you'll reap the rewards.

So, with all of that said, what comprises a healthy breakfast?

1. Protein

Foods that are rich in protein can help with balancing the blood sugar levels in the body, so you end up craving much less food throughout the day. This is a deterrent to incessant snacking! Hard-boiled and poached eggs are both ideal dishes when it comes to breakfast. Both would also provide you with enough energy to use until lunch time comes. Yoghurt is also another popular breakfast item. If you want a bit more protein in it, adding in your favourite protein-rich nuts or protein powder should do the trick.

2. Carbohydrates

Back when you were still in school, the teacher would often tell you about the go, grow, and glow foods. Carbohydrates are included in the "go" section which means that these types of foods are capable of giving you energy which you can then use to achieve "go" for the tasks and activities without getting tired easily.

What else can you add to your daily breakfast if you don't have much time in the mornings? Well, there's oatmeal, fruits, whole-grain bread, cereals, peanut butter and smoothies. However, do keep in mind that there are also certain food items which you shouldn't have. This would include all types of processed foods such as hotdog, sausage, and bacon.

Give more importance to this meal because this will keep you going throughout the day. As much as possible, make a weekly plan so as not to forget the foods required for a healthy breakfast.

Start Getting Physically Fit

Exercise, but only do so during the mornings. This is because doing it at night can give you trouble sleeping. Keep in mind that exercise is meant to get your blood going and your energy to its maximum. It would be pretty hard to wind down after that. You must continue to do it every morning to prepare your soul, mind, and body for the tasks and activities for the whole day. Once you have had a good night's sleep, you are now ready to start your day right.

Doing some simple exercise in the morning would wake you up far better than coffee ever would. Jogging around the house and doing simple stretches are both great to get you warmed up. If you're not the type to exercise regularly, try not to overexert yourself out of excitement. With this, it is important to pace yourself. Remember, you're healing! You wouldn't want to injure yourself in the process.

To motivate yourself in doing exercises every morning, here are a few reasons why you need to do it:

Regular exercise is equal to a good amount of sleep.

Working out, much like sleeping or taking a shot of your favourite coffee, is capable of keeping you alert and awake for most of the day. You might even avoid the need to take a siesta, especially during the early hours of the afternoon when lethargy tends to visit.

<u>It boosts your concentration.</u>

A few minutes of workout will make you more productive. It energises your body and mind, so you have more strength and clear thinking to accomplish the tasks needed for work or school.

<u>It helps with increasing the speed of your metabolism.</u>

If you want to lower the number of calories in your body, you will need to exercise regularly, and go to the gym several times. However, you can prevent this build up by doing a few minutes of exercise in the morning. In doing so, you are helping your body become better when it comes to calorie-burning. What this means is that if you end up eating a bit more than usual throughout the day, your body is more efficient at burning everything up and turning it to energy. And what does more energy mean? MORE POWER, MORE STRENGTH and BETTER PRODUCTIVITY.

It makes your heart stronger.

You may have had your heart broken, but trust me when I say that it is far more resilient than most people give it credit for. It will continue its job despite your heartaches so you should do the same. Show your heart some love by doing cardio exercises. This increases blood flow to the body and helps prevent the build-up of plaque in the heart as well as the arteries. Strengthen your heart; it will undoubtedly thank you for it.

Now, that you have the motivation to do a few stretches and movements, you need to follow these simple rules for morning exercise:

1. Do it right after waking up.

Do not procrastinate as doing so would welcome thoughts that say, "Don't do it." So, right after you got out of bed, do your warm-ups then proceed with your morning exercise. Push yourself if you're feeling lazy about it—remind yourself why you're doing this in the first place. Self-empowerment is key.

2. Make your movements big and exciting.

Morning exercises are usually short and only consist of easy workout routines. That said, it also shouldn't be boring. If you want to, turn your routine into something similar to dance, put on some great music and sweat all that negativity out of your body. Should you prefer quieter exercises, however, then yoga should provide you with a good challenge.

3. It should be done for a few minutes only.

You do not want to overdo yourself by exercising for hours. It can be done for 5 to 15 minutes each day and may include a few easy stretches and cardio movements. It depends on your own needs so don't forget to consider that.

4. Establish aesthetic goals.

Revenge body. You have heard of it before, and it is currently the motivation for people everywhere to start getting healthy. However, always do things specifically because you want to be better—not because you want to get even with an ex. Do things for yourself and not because you're trying to impress someone else. If having a smaller waist would help you be more confident, then do it!

Morning exercises might be hard to do at first, but always try to identify its advantage; there's plenty and not just for your body, too. A few minutes of working out is a great thing to add to your everyday routine.

Get Enough Sleep (Go to bed early, Wake up early)

Many people think that a good morning routine starts when you wake up. It begins the night before you go to sleep. Studies have shown that the ideal amount of time required for the average person to sleep is seven to nine hours. If you sleep below or beyond that time, there will be negative effects. That is why, if you want to be productive in the morning, you should planning the night before.

What happens if you don't get enough rest? Here are the negative effects of lack of sleep:

1. Your body will gain weight.

Sleep deprivation causes the body to produce hormones called ghrelin. It increases the appetite so you will crave for more food during the day. That is why people who lack sleep are more prone to obesity.

2. Your mind will not work perfectly.

Researchers found out that people who sleep less than six hours a day experience anxiety and depression. Before bedtime, people tend to reflect on and evaluate events that happened during the day. If you think and worry a lot, the thoughts will keep on coming until you realised that it's already late in the evening. Clear your mind as much as possible for a few minutes or hours before you go to bed.

3. Your immune system will be weak.

When you sleep, your immune system produces proteins called cytokines. It encourages sleep. So, if you are sleep deprived, there will be a decrease in the production of these protective proteins. You end up becoming more prone to illnesses and viruses.

There are more negative effects of lack of sleep, but these three are the main points. Sometimes, it can be especially hard for a person to follow a sleep schedule. It may be because of their work or activities during the day, but there is always something that can be done about it. Time management is important. You just need to be disciplined and strict about it. To help you develop a proper sleeping pattern, here are some tips on how you can sleep earlier and better at night:

1. When you feel tired, do not hesitate to doze off.

Sometimes, a person just needs to listen to their body. It will tell you what to do to keep healthy. So, if you keep on yawning and feel that your body is already tired, and then sleep. It is what you need at the moment. If you do not follow what your body is trying to tell you, there's a greater chance that you'll experience more illnesses in the future.

2. set a "before bedtime" habit.

Think of the things that make you sleepy. Taking a shower, reading a book, or listening to classical music are some examples of how you can encourage your body to rest. Decide on one activity and push yourself to do it before the time you set for sleeping. Avoid things that will just keep you more awake like drinking coffee or updating social media.

3. Set the time when to sleep and when to wake up.

Determine what time you are going to wake up in the morning, then subtract 8 hours from it. That is the hour at which you need to sleep at night. For example, you need to go to work at 8 in the morning. So, the ideal time to wake up is at 6 AM. If you subtract 8 hours in the clock, you get 10 PM.

If you have already identified your sleeping schedule, follow it with discipline. Do not make excuses or contradict it. You will be the one benefitting from it after all.

4. Write down reasons why you need to sleep early.

Write down the things you need to do the next day. This will serve as reminders of the tasks you need to accomplish. They become your motivation and something you can look forward to the following day. If there are no scheduled activities, make your own. They will give you excitement and inspiration to rest for the whole night.

5. Reward yourself.

According to experts, it will take you at least 30 days to establish a new habit. So during that month, be diligent and patient in following your routine until it is no longer hard for you to go to sleep early. Treat yourself to good food or a nice movie for a job well done.

Be Happy Every day

Do you want to be happy every day? Love yourself first. If you have already accepted who you are and what you can do, you can be confident in all the ways. You will gain more positive thinking in everything you do. Good things will continually come your way. What has happened in the past would become nothing more than an afterthought; something that you experienced and has taught you how to become a better person. Nothing more than a bump in the road to becoming successful.

But does success equal happiness? Not quite. Happiness is something you choose and practice every single day. Here are a few tips:

Do one act of kindness a day. Helping other people is not a burden. In fact, after performing an act of kindness that brightens another person's day, you will absorb some of that positivity for yourself. Happiness becomes more real if you share it with another.

Learn to forgive. It may be yourself or people close to you. The people who have done you wrong and caused you grief. Forgive yourself for making bad decisions in your life and move on. It will lighten the baggage you have been carrying for a long time.

Face your fears. Everyone has one, and not facing it will result in more fears. It will affect your everyday routine and your health. You will get stuck in your life because it will bring you down. So, face it and be stronger!

Dream big. This is not a bad thing. You can choose to dream bigger things, and in doing so, you might even achieve more than what you expected to. If you are inspired and have the motivation, you can reach them.

HAPPINESS CHECKLIST:

- *Get up early.*

- *Remind yourself of your life's purpose.*

- *Exercise regularly.*

- *Eat healthy foods.*

- *Get some sunlight.*

- *Be confident in everything you do.*

- *Absorb only the positive energies around you.*

- *Find new motivation every day.*

- *Move on from failures and heartaches.*

- *Have something to look forward to.*

- *Learn something new.*

- *Be grateful even for small things.*

- *Make someone happy, too.*

That is just a simple list you can use every day. But, you can also make your own and add more items. There are just a lot of things you can do to be happy.

Chapter 6 - Moving Forward

With all the tips and advice written in the previous chapters, you'll realise that moving on is not as easy as it may seem. You have to invest time, strength, and determination to achieve it. Most people who have gone through a bad breakup will only recover after he or she has decided to stop looking back and instead, continue moving forward — accepting the pain and reality of their situation made "moving on" possible. You can, too.

In the end, you'll look back at this bad memory, and it won't hurt anymore. The only thing left would be the lessons you learned from it. To complete the process, you should also be able to:

Creating Your Happiness

First of all, you should know what hinders you from creating your happiness. Sometimes you feel responsible for the happiness of others. You feel guilty when you say "no" or refuse people especially those who are very close to you. But when you do that, you forget that you should have done something for yourself first.

Here are questions that you can ask yourself to know how you can create your happiness:

- What makes you happy?

Problems are inevitable. Sometimes, it can make you think negatively about life. And most of the time, those problems are not that big as you think they are. Look at the picture and remind yourself of your own goals.

Write down the little things that make you happy. It can be the songs you hear on the radio, the messages and letters you got from your friends. It can even be the food that you eat at your favourite buffet restaurant. You will soon realise that you do not need grand things to achieve happiness. Just be grateful for the small things you have and the simple moments you experience.

- What are you good at?

You cannot please everyone. Your parents, relatives, and friends have their expectations for you. But sometimes, those expectations do not match yours. When this happens, prioritise yourself. Even if their expectations seem more significant than yours, do not be pressured. You can lose your self if you keep on trying to live up to other people's expectations. It will not help you gain confidence in yourself and your own decisions in life.

Maximise your strengths and improve on your weaknesses. If you are good at music, make the most of it and be a great musician. Focus on the things you shine at and do your best to achieve your full potential.

- Who is your inspiration?

Knowing what you want to achieve in life and having an inspiration gives you more purpose. It makes you see the bigger picture of what your dreams look like when you have succeeded in them.

But, you should also choose your role models carefully. Find someone who has made it to the top by their hard work and tries to take away as much as you can learn from them. Remember, if they made it then you most certainly can as well.

- What do you need to let go of?

What hinders you from moving forward? If you're joining a marathon, will you bring a heavy bag with you? Will you wear heavy clothes like pants and thick jackets? No. Because those things will just slow you down. You will get tired easily having to carry those unnecessary items. It is the same thing with the marathon of life towards achieving your happiness, goals, and dreams. The lighter your baggage, the better.

- What keeps you from doing something?

Do you feel that you are not good enough? Are you scared of the criticisms you might get from other people? Fear is probably what keeps you from doing what you want to do.

You won't get anywhere if you're too scared to make the first step.

Remember that even the most successful people did not achieve their dreams right away. They experienced a lot of failures along the way too. But their secret is that they kept on trying. Pushing themselves even after they have fallen. They are not scared to try again even if they have failed a million times. Courage is the key. Trust yourself and have faith in what you're capable of.

- What do you need to change?

Doing what you love should make you feel happy, not stressed. If you feel like you are always in a bad mood, impatient, or running out of time, it is time to make some changes.

Evaluate your schedule every day. You should have proper time management and organizational skills. With this, you won't need to cram or be pressured whilst trying to finish the things you need to do.

- Who are your real friends?

Acknowledge the people who are always there with you regardless of the situation you're in. Good and bad, they didn't leave your side. The people who, when you have a problem, you can always call to receive some encouragement. The same ones you can also call to celebrate success. Avoid taking them for granted.

Choose friends that will understand you even if you are busy and will also make time for you if you need them. Do not forget to be the same kind of friend for them, too. Surrounding yourself with good friends will encourage you to move forward with confidence.

- Whose opinion matters?

Friends listen well to your problems but if more significant problems arise, who do you ask? People who are older are more experienced in life. These people can include your parents, grandparents, aunts, uncles, or even a mentor. People who have experienced plenty and have also collected much of their wisdom through it. Develop a good relationship with them. If you don't agree with some of their opinions on the matter, that's fine. It is still important to listen for you never know what insight they might be able to provide you with.

- How can you be confident?

You may have noticed that some people are very confident in everything they do. But everyone experiences fear and insecurity too. No exceptions. Their secret is that they know how to handle and deal with those negative thoughts.

If you are scared of facing a lot of people, do it more often. Face your fears and keep doing it until you have overcome them. It may take a while but remember the goals that you want to reach. Keep being inspired and motivated all the time and this will make you a more confident person.

These are questions that you should ask yourself to move forward with your life after a divorce or breakup. You may have been through a setback, but you can always heal from the heartache.

As you continue with your life, take with you the lessons you have learned from every heartbreak and hardship. Eventually, you will find

that true love that you have wished
for.

Conclusion

Thanks again for taking the time to purchase Self-love and Personal Transformation: Get Back Your Confidence and Learn to Love Yourself after a Relationship Breakup.

You should now have a good understanding of how you can move on from heartbreak or hardship and be able to turn something negative into a positive that would enable you to become a much better person.

About the Author

Stirling De Cruz-Coleridge published author, philanthropist and entrepreneur.

Books by Stirling De Cruz-Coleridge:

- *Live Your Life with Success, Good Habits and Love: 45 Highly Effective Habits of Successful People*

- *Success, Happiness, Power, and Money: How to Make Your Life Awesome in 15 Ways*

- *Emotional Healing & Personal Transformation: 7 Ways on How to Handle a Breakup When You Still Love Them*

- *Powerful, Motivational Success Habits and Personal Transformation: 10 Effective Ways to Create Self Confidence and an Awesome Life*

- *Learning and Memory: How to Use Advanced Strategies & Techniques to Remember More, Learn More, Accelerate Your Brain Power & How to Avoid Memory Deficit in Later Life*

- *Menopausal Brain Fog Memory: Strategies to Help Women Think Straight and Cope Better in the Workplace*

OVERCOME DEPRESSION & STOP YOUR MISERY NOW

Guide for Increasing Self-Esteem, Overcoming Depression, Anxiety, Sadness and Living Your Life.

ABOUT THIS BOOK:

You know how depressed, anxious and sad you feel at times or all the time? You don't want to feel this way but how can you stop it? The book contains a multiple plan for overcoming depression and anxiety or sadness. It can teach you how to deal with many things. Find out strategies that can change your life. Master coping techniques, skills and tools on how they will benefit you.

Have you not noticed or felt like the entire world is changing? Is something going on around us that we don't know about? There is so much happening around us these days, quite horrible things going wrong, that it is so difficult to be sure about anything these days. There doesn't seem to be much certainty about anything. So why do we feel so down and depressed, anxious and sad? Everyone has all kinds of reasons; personal tragedies, that it's so hard to keep up with it and in the midst of it all, we need to find, calm, peace and happiness once again.

Does one size fit all? No, it doesn't, there is more than one solution to your problems. Find out the multiple ways you can overcome depression and stop your misery now. This guide tackles depression from several different angles, not one. It will help increase self-esteem, assist you in overcoming depression, anxiety and sadness so that you can start living your life today.

OVERCOME DEPRESSION & STOP YOUR MISERY NOW

Guide for Increasing Self-Esteem, Overcoming Depression, Anxiety, Sadness and Living Your Life

Stirling De Cruz-Coleridge

Disclaimer

This document is geared towards providing exact and reliable information in regards to the topic and issue covered. The publication is sold with the idea that the publisher is not required to render an accounting, officially permitted, or otherwise, qualified services. If advice is necessary, legal or professional, a practised individual in the profession should be ordered.

- From a Declaration of Principles which was accepted and approved equally by a Committee of the American Bar Association and a

Under no circumstances will any legal responsibility or blame be held against the publisher for any reparation, damages, or monetary loss due to the information herein, either directly or indirectly.

Respective authors own all copyrights not held by the publisher.

The information herein is offered for informational purposes solely and is universal as so. The presentation of the information is without a contract or any type of guarantee assurance.

The trademarks that are used are without any consent, and the publication of the trademark is without permission or backing by the trademark owner. All trademarks and brands within this book are for clarifying purposes only and are owned by the owners themselves, not affiliated with this document.

If you suffer from any form of clinical depression illness, it is advisable that you seek the advice of a medical professional.

Introduction

Have you not noticed or felt like the entire world is changing? Is something going on around us that we don't know about? There is so much happening around us these days, quite horrible things going wrong, that it is so difficult to be sure about anything these days. There doesn't seem to be much certainty about anything. Why do we feel so down and depressed? Everyone has all kinds of reasons; personal tragedies that it's so hard to keep up with it. In the midst of it all, we need to find, calm, peace and happiness again, but how?

I first want to share with you my journey. Back in 2009, I was working in a job I hated, and I was unhappy. I was becoming overwhelmed with my workload, the people I worked with were awful and backstabbing too, I was also 45 pounds overweight, and I had a string of failed relationships behind me. I had severe social anxiety, and the friends I kept and the family relations I had were not very helpful. I had a limited social life, and when I did go out, it was an endurance test. I had nothing in common with the company I was in. It was a deep, dark place for many years and my depression made me feel nothing but self-pity almost 24/7 hours per day. My mind would not shut off.

On most days, I couldn't even find the inclination to get out of my bed. I drowned in my sorrows by drinking alcohol excessively five nights a week and eating junk food about 2-3 times per week. I was heading into a vicious downward spiral. It was either sink or swim. Besides that, I lost a dear loved one; my rock someone so significant to me and it was painstaking because I lost a loved one through a terminal illness.

This meant I had to be strong for others in my family. I was not able to grieve like a regular person would because other people were fortunate enough to have others to rely on in great times of need. The family friends I had were not supportive and were quite prepared to abandon me when I needed their support. I have just about touched on the surface of what I went through in my life, to be honest, I could write a book on it.

Nevertheless, I decided to swim; I had not come this far in my achievements in life and the rotten things that had happened to me. I am writing this contently, in my attempt to share with you my knowledge on what it takes to overcome depression as a result of situational disasters.

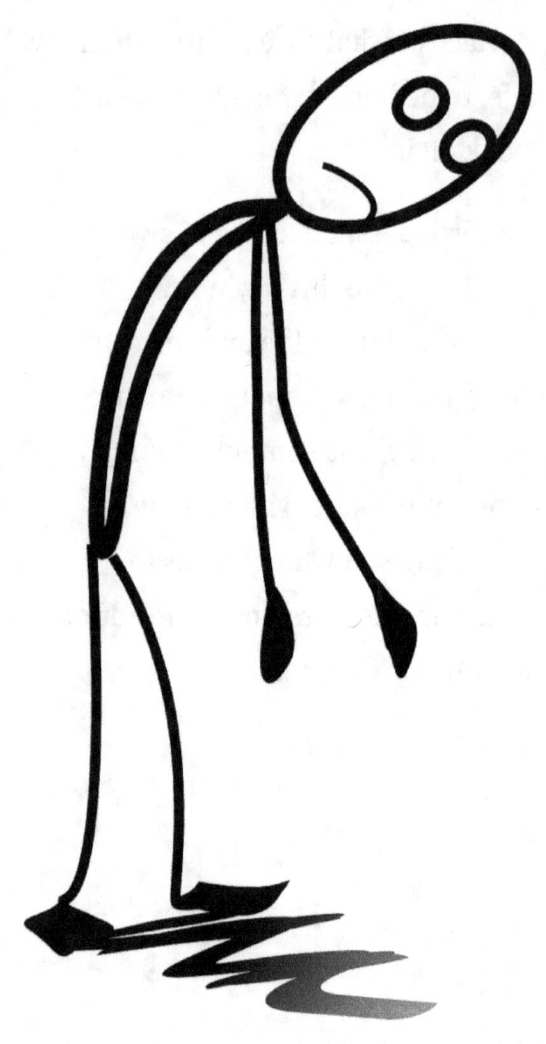

Please accept it from me. First of all, I want you to know that no matter where you stand at this present moment in your life, it is possible to make changes. Don't give in because you can live your desires and do amazing things in this worldwide too. If you are reading this book, you can get back on the right track. This book is going to offer you multiple methods and tips that you can use to steadily climb out from the pits of depression to the elevations of joy and hope.

I can not tell you it will certainly not be simple, yet I can assure you it's well worth it. Whatever you desire can be just around the corner. If you dedicate and devote time to your self-development and pledge to yourself to never surrender and give up, then you will undoubtedly conquer and do extraordinary things, and be a motivation to others.

If you do not have a belief in your ability to overcome depression or anxiety, then that's okay, since this book will undoubtedly provide you with the hope and motivation that you will need. I'm right here to offer you a helping hand because I understand that none of us can do this alone — my support and love is heading out to you. I know you will certainly make it with this.

So now let's explore what it's going to take, shall we?

Nature vs Nurture

From experience and research, I'm convinced that depression is entirely internal. Nevertheless, outside variables can play a huge role in identifying your inner landscape, atmosphere (your thoughts and attitudes). Positioning the blame on these external conditions is easy to do. However, it should be circumvented at all costs, especially as we know that circumstances and situations are always changing. So you need a firm foundation, to begin with, right?

So instead, you need to take full responsibility for your current events as well as understand that you have unconsciously created them. You might not have yearned for them, however via a series of ideas and choices; you have brought them into your life. This implies you are additionally in charge of transforming them if that's what you desire. Some external things that might be having an adverse influence on you could be friends, family members, and your work; the TV shows and films you watch and some of the songs you listen to, perhaps the food you eat, or the tidiness of your room even. The list can go on and on. However, these are just some of the significant things you need to recognise.

I will certainly go into a couple of them in more detail later, however, for now, I would like you to look at your life from an objective viewpoint and also try to see whether a few of the above things may be holding you back. Possibly your work may be demanding, as well as you do not appreciate it whatsoever, or perhaps you have the propensity to watch terrible flicks and TV programmes. Maybe you have friends or family that aren't very encouraging of you or likely your home is a mess and also by just checking it out, it makes you feel impoverished and poor in spirit. Whatever it is, it's essential that you confess this to yourself that some things do need transforming. Don't fret about changing anything right now. Merely understanding the problem is enough. Understanding is the foundation and structure of favourable modification. When you begin being truthful with yourself and also begin to notice the areas of your life that are triggering you with unfavourable emotions like sadness, misery or anger, for example, your life will typically start to enhance. Remember, rejection guarantees stagnancy — awareness warranties development.

When I started my trip of self-development many years ago, the first considerable thing that changed was my circle of close friends. I quit socialising with a whole lot of individuals I used to be very close to. It occurred by itself without me needing to do much about it. I was enhancing myself so quickly that old close friends naturally fell away and were soon left behind. We had no more things in common. This can happen when you work with people, for example, you start to socialise with them a lot, you go out drinking and once the job ends, so do the friendships; most of which were developed in social drinking circles after work, in bars after a hard day.

Over time, I was concentrated more on becoming active and happy, while they were still doing the same old things they had been doing for years. I understood that I might not manage to mix with certain individuals that didn't have similar goals as I did. It was nothing versus them. However, I recognised the relevance of putting myself in the very best atmosphere possible. They claim you end up being like the five or six people you spend the most times with, and I have discovered that to be so real.

I'm telling you this since, from my experience, I've been concerned to see that the first thing that can hold people back from attaining their objectives and also jumping on the path to a better life is their circle of buddies. Sometimes, no one wants you to be successful or happy as if they want you to remain like them. The painful truth is that you will most likely need to cut some individuals out of your life if you desire far better things for yourself.

You cannot afford to hang out with negative individuals if you wish to live a positive life. If you are fortunate enough, after that, you may find some new accommodating and motivating friends. Keep those people close, but take into consideration getting rid of or significantly minimising the quantity of time you invest with the individuals who aren't delighted or doing much with their lives. You will become like the individuals you hang around with for sure, and this can impact on your mind and feelings of despair and depression.

Their behaviours, as well as tendencies, will rub off on you swiftly. Who wants to listen to their gossip and moaning about trivial things? On my journey, I've invested a great deal of time alone for this reason. It's continuously a much better concept to be alone than to be with negative individuals. And also being alone offers you an excellent opportunity to discover how to like yourself more, which is vital for living a happy and fulfilling life.

Every little thing that you take in from the outside atmosphere that you allow to enter into your mind and body unconsciously comes to be a component of your interior atmosphere, known as *introjection.* Memories get stored, good and bad energy taken in, and influences and perspectives of especially others can become engrained in your mind. An example of this might be adopting other people's values and attitudes.

Everything from your workplace location; to the kind of music you pay attention to, influences your thoughts as well as attitudes. Considering that your thoughts determine the quality of your life and your degree of happiness, you would be smart to re-evaluate your life as well as choose what is offering you something good or useful as well as what is not. If something doesn't feel ideal or makes you feel negative, after that it needs to be prevented. This process requires time and requires recognition, yet it will have a significant effect on your life.

Familiarising your outer atmosphere is vital. However, I believe that knowingly forming your life from the inside out is much more effective.

Since your thoughts have led to the decisions that got you to where you are today, concentrating on improving your ideas will guarantee you finish up in a better place than you are right now.

You did the best thing when you searched for a book like this one, but it was a thought that drove you to it in the first place. Individuals often tend to think that whatever happens "happens, or that's life" when in truth everything happens "for a reason." Adjust your ideas, transform your life. You will undoubtedly discover that your outside atmosphere immediately transforms as your internal atmosphere adjusts. I have seen this to be real for myself, as well as I have researched many other successful people that all claim the very same thing. Change begins from within. This does not imply that you overlook making changes to your external environment if you can, like looking for a better job for example. It indicates that most of your time spent improving on yourself must be concentrated from within.

The following stage will explain precisely how to shape your inner self for optimum success as well as happiness.

Mindfulness: The Basis of Positive Change

For somebody that is feeling depressed, self-contemplation, as well as self-analysis, is a must. There is frequently the tendency to intend to stay clear of problems as well as repress emotions out of a concern of confronting and facing them, but this should be prevented. You have to agree to confront any of your internal demons to have any chance of clearing them and moving on from them. Even more so, should you avoid them, the much more profound as well as deeper they will go, the more difficult they become to remove later on down the line, believe me.

Repressed emotions influence the body in a hugely recognisable way. They trigger tension in the muscular tissues of the body, which can bring about persistent stress and anxiety, frustration, hypertension, extreme anxiousness, and quite often transpire into a disease. It is crucial that you muster up the nerve to go within yourself and deal with the underlying reasons for your current condition or situation. It can be terrifying at first. However, it is very much needed. It's not so weak when you become aware that you are not your thoughts. You are just the momentary proprietor of ideas, which implies you can regulate and control your ideas, thoughts and opinions, not vice versa. Having unfavourable views does not indicate you are an evildoer. It just demonstrates that you have momentarily lost touch with who you are. And that you indeed are a person who is far greater than who you presently believe you indeed are.

Beneath all those adverse ideas is a stunning person with unlimited potential. You might not see it currently, yet I promise that you will when you conquer this and also discover how to be happy once again. As I mentioned, when I was in the process of overcoming my extreme anxiety years ago I spent a substantial amount of time alone, reading and learning. I'm an introvert by nature, so it was what I chose quite naturally. If you are an introvert, you do have a minor advantage. Although I think introverts are much more prone to depression because they introspect a lot, often undertaking a detailed examination of their thoughts, feelings and motives anyway, but I believe it more probable that introverts conquer their depression.

Getting rid of depression requires a great deal of introspection as well as self-analysis, which as I said introverts also do naturally. This is, so they tend to overcome their problems much quicker. On the other hand, extroverted people tend to look outside of themselves for their answers, not realising that which troubles them from within. Due to the nature of extroverted people, they might have an added problem resolving inner conflicts and issues. At the same time, they are proficient at briefly forgetting their troubles due to their sense of escapism or outgoing, social nature. While introverts often sit or lie about and stew in their emotions; often leading into a descending spiral of anxiety and depression. Both have their advantages as well as challenges. However, the real message that I wish to convey here is the importance of facing your problems instead of preventing or avoiding them. And also by that, I mean looking within you first.

You may think your problem exists outside, worldwide somewhere; however, you will certainly never be able to produce long-term modifications in your life unless you first change from the inside. You may be able to fix a broken partnership momentarily, but if you didn't do any of the needed internal jobs within yourself, the very same relationship issues will at some point appear once again. Or perhaps, you might have the ability to obtain some short-term joy by going on holiday or by changing jobs; however, that happiness will not last if you did not change your internal setting that is your thoughts and ideas or your perspectives towards life.

You can relocate to the loveliest place in the world, yet you still have to take your mind and your whole body with you, right? If you do not discover that you need to go within yourself first and alter your ideas, then nothing will positively transform. If you read this entire book, after that you will be mindful that something in your life requires adjusting. It's an excellent indication that you are reviewing this because that shows you are concerned, and you accept some responsibility for your current situation in buying this book.

Some people have way too much pride to confess that they need to transform. Fortunately, that is not you. Now, you need to go a little much deeper and attempt to reveal the original cause of your anxiety or depression. You may currently have a good idea, but it's essential that you get as specific as possible because that will undoubtedly enable you to re-contextualise things as well as see them in a more favourable light. The next area will certainly explain a necessary process for you to discover the concealed blocks stopping you from living the life you deserve, right now.

Self-examination and Analysis

For me, the only way to solve anything for myself is to go within and figure out the thoughts and mindsets that were regulating my responses as well as interpretations of events and conditions around me. I recognised that the problem was with my perception, feelings and beliefs, so my primary purpose was to expose the details and ideas that were the cause of my long-time suffering. I acknowledged that when I found them, I can start to let them go and replace them with more favourable ideas that helped me far better in coping.

The method I started with was with innovative self-expression via writing and particularly poetry. Verses allowed me to express my thoughts in a creative way that I could feel pleased with myself. Also though my thoughts were mostly negative, I did not feel so bad regarding them when I expressed them in the form of art. It was a real recovery for me to get my thoughts out onto paper. It was something that made me genuinely delighted at that point in my life. I firmly think that everyone that is experiencing depression can benefit significantly from expressing themselves through writing and art in some form or other. Look at all the famous artists we have over the years, those brilliant geniuses

produced works of art from
expressing themselves is my point.

Somehow when I got things down on
paper, the whole process of writing
or composing in it was quite healing.
But what makes creating incredibly
useful is the truth that it produces
and self-awareness. Drawing up your
thoughts enables you to see them in
concrete form, wherefore otherwise,
they are merely ideas. Quite often
some of my negative thoughts didn't
appear so bad when written on
paper. When those thoughts run out
of your head, you suddenly can no
more relate to them the same way
you did before when they were
floating about in your head. So,
instead of evaluating and
condemning yourself for your awful

evil thoughts, you realise that they are merely words, and also words can be transformed. Let us look at the next stage.

Journal

I honestly encourage you to begin or adopt a journaling technique soon. Try freehand writing for a minimum of 5-10 minutes per day without modifying or censoring yourself. Write what enters into your mind. Spill your guts out if needs are. Nobody is going to see or review it except you, so you can be entirely honest with yourself and allow your personal, darkest ideas to rise and surface here. From there, they can be released onto paper through the pen in your hand, and you will be freed of one burden after another every time you write. I want to motivate and encourage every person to write in a journal every day if possible. Let silly or negative thoughts and headlines run across your forehead or your mind like news Teletext and then jot them down in your journal. Don't react to any of those thoughts write them down. I had to do this before I was trained as a counsellor for counselling training by the way. We had to be done to clear out our minds first before counselling anyone! So it does work.

However, you specifically need to do this if you are feeling down or depressed or battling with negative emotions. It's unbelievable to see the change that occurs just from this one simple method. Begin this today if you can. If it helps, get an exceptional leather-bound journal or something vibrant that is pleasing for you to look at each day. Get excited about it especially have a place of retreat to go to and pour out your heart into it, your thoughts from the day and any troubles. This is your life nevertheless, and this is one step in the right direction of a far brighter future. Journaling itself is a powerful tool, but I have a few pointers that will aid you to make it even much more transformative.

Once you have written your entry for the day, re-read what you have created as well as try to point out any unfavourable thoughts and ideas you might have jotted down. Now, choose one of them and try to re-write it or *reframe* it at the bottom of the note page. After that, you are most likely to re-frame that declaration to make it sound slightly more positive. This is the way you will turn on your own, from a pessimist to an optimist, an adverse thinker to a positive one, which will make all the difference in your life.

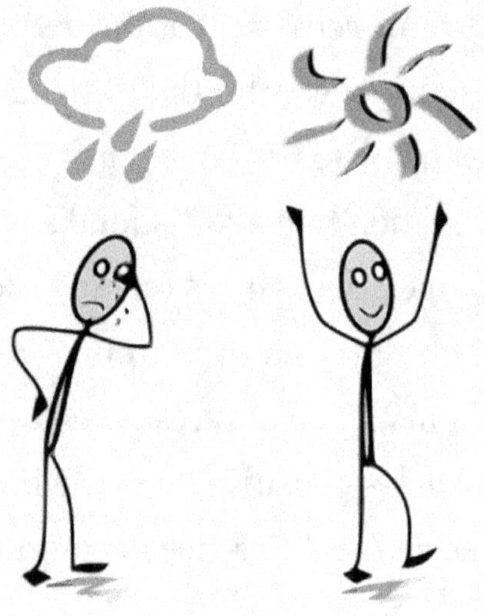

Reframing

This simple technique can be used to turn a negative statement or question with a negative frame of reference, into one which has a far more positive value and tone to it. It's used as a form of self-protection for example when you are in the company of negative naysayers or negative thinkers, particularly those who are more likely to thrive on any self-criticism or worries you may share with them. You will notice in the following examples, how by reframing your sentences, you can help yourself think more positively and at the same time setting a perkier tone to a conversational exchange, therefore, lessening any

chance of being loaded up with
moans or put-downs.

An example would be:

"What a never-ending queue! I'm going to go insane standing here wasting my time, isn't it a disgraceful service?"

But instead, you could say, *"This is a long queue, so at least I have 5-10 minutes uninterrupted time to sort out my thoughts or switch-off for a while, perhaps have a chat or, check my mobile phone."*

Another example, if you had a bad day and wrote, *"Nothing went well for me today. It felt like others were against me, and nothing seems to work out the way I want it to."*

Once you have created this statement at the bottom of the page, and write below it, compose something like,

"Today could have been a bad day, but I know that there are better days ahead. My future is hopeful, and I will not allow a bad day ruin my state of mind."

Circle this latter positive statement. Hey presto! You have effectively reframed a negative thought into a more favourable one, and you are currently one step better off to become the happy, confident, enthusiastic person you desire to be.

You see, you always have the choice of exactly how you wish to consider things and their outcome. A negative scenario is just adverse in the eyes of the person that decides to see it that way, by doing this. You can always choose to transform a bad situation into a positive one. It takes time and a lot of practice too. However, it is well worth the preliminary initiative because positive thoughts bring positive results — your joy is directly associated with the number of optimistic ideas that you adopt.

To beat depression fast and to experience significant amounts of joy, your primary purpose needs to continually be to consider the essential things in your life in an extra positive light. Truth is very subjective.

Misfortune

A tragedy to one person can be a blessing to another. It's not always about the circumstance itself but instead your perception of it. I am not suggesting that bad things don't happen, they do, and it can feel terrible. But how can we genuinely handle the seemingly unfavourable events that are an unavoidable part of life?

- *People do die*
- *People develop ill health*
- *Friendship connections do end*
- *Accidents happen*
- *Job loss happens*
- *Some have little or no money*
- *Anyone can become homeless*
- *cars do get damaged*
- *marriages and partnerships can break up*
- *some eat to self-soothe and then pile on weight*

Some of these are hard facts there is no denying it. And a great deal more can be added to this list in the shape of other events that the majority of people will see as being 'tragic' or 'regrettable' incidents. They are, and I am not lessening any of them by any means. Instead, I am emphasising here that it is not what happens but, how you view or perceive it.

I have an easy suggestion or solution to these issues, and that is, always seek the lesson learned in all of them. All adverse situations sometimes hold a concealed message, a gem or hidden treasure for you, somewhere along the line. Many people's instant response to unfortunate events is to over-dramatise it even more or state, "*Oh dear, how awful*" or "*What bad luck.*" The majority of people instantly look for the issue instead of the solution. I'll inform you about something here, and that is that life becomes a lot more attractive when you search for the good in all things, the silver lining and, there is nothing more significant than a matter of selection or choice.

You might be automatically conditioned to look for the misfortune instead of the lesson behind the tragedy, but that's fairly typical as well as it is why I have shown you and a lot more people about the journaling, reframing and processing exercise.

When you start reframing all your negative thoughts and ideas, your entire world will slowly begin to improve. When you can construct desirable thinking behaviour patterns, life often has a habit of exercising more favour in your direction. Even if it doesn't, you will undoubtedly be searching for the beauty in it and therefore, you will find it.

Even in the midst of depression, it can be tough to discover the lesson in it. You probably will not do so right away. It may take time to see the incredible true blessing that it is; however, I encourage you to begin looking for the positives from now. My anxiety was my biggest blessing since it allowed me to focus and concentrate on bettering myself. If it had not been for my depression, I would probably still be living a sub-par life. I did not see just how my depression was a real blessing until well over ten years ago after it declined considerably. However, today it is more evident to me. Tears of pleasure and thankfulness often roll down my cheeks when I stop to think of all the battles I've conquered.

I guarantee you that you will review your current situation or battle as well as feel the same as I did. The lesson's hidden at the minute, yet your work is to reveal it and to turn this battle into a tiny stepping stone for your greater achievements to come.

At the beginning of self-contemplation and self-analysis, a whole lot of unfavourable ideas and emotions will begin to surface. This might be uncomfortable at first; however, it is necessary for your individual growth.

Dedicate to writing in a journal each day; you will see great progression gradually. Having the honesty to confess the visibility of unfavourable as well as unsafe thoughts is a significant action in and of itself. You have gone beyond the phase of denial as well as victimhood and repositioned yourself right into courage and self-commitment. At this phase, your healing virtually assured.

The speed at which you recoup will rely on your capability to surrender your issues as well as select an extra favourable focus. The entire procedure will be a lot simpler if you can come to a degree of understanding as well as self-acceptance. I'll cover this area in more detail in the next section.

Self Approval: Let Go of Your Problems

Approval is a vital step in the procedure of transcending negativity and rising to a degree of pleasure as well as fulfilment. At a level of negativity, making adverse decisions that have negative effects is very typical, because choices at this level often result from psychological placements not based on rational thinking or in some cases, morality. At the level of negativity, it is effortless to be entrapped in a vicious cycle of negative decisions based on wrong reasoning that leads to negative consequences, therefore strengthening and reinforcing the unfavourable attitude in yourself generally.

Remember that it just appears so that it can be fixed. In the past, you most likely weren't extremely familiar with the particular thoughts that were causing your unfavourable feelings, and so you have most likely been placing a great deal of blame on yourself. When you end up being much more conscious, you will not feel the requirement to be so tough on yourself. You will undoubtedly see that your ideas do not define you. They occur *automatically* as a result of your past conditioning.

Today you recognise your thoughts and also understand that they can be changed and they no longer have to control you. Now you can take back your power and forgive yourself for not being aware of this in the past. You could not alter anything at that time because you did not have the expertise and also the understanding to do so. You can kick back understanding that you can exercise optimal control over your life. The following area will instruct you just how to do so.

Psychological Reprogramming and Positive Momentum

The mind is an incredible device for processing and navigating the world. However, it additionally has many problems. The brain is conveniently predisposed to its surrounding as well as subtle instructions and also images. One should be extremely mindful in the world and prevent getting entrapped in a cycle of negative thoughts. It's entirely reasonable to experience severe 'lows' in life, and also it is continuously for our highest good sometimes, as long as we take a look at it as a discovering lesson. Some people, however, come to be stuck in their thoughts and sensations of lethargy and self-pity.

This keeps them caught in negativity. Getting rid of the negativity is just feasible with a readiness to see things differently and to look for help from others or professionals. You're doing fantastic if you are reading this book. It indicates you have kept an open mind as well as want to find out more. I applaud you for that, and I am happy about the possibility to reveal my knowledge to you. I have gotten rid of the depths of depression and extreme stress and anxiety, and I did it mostly through the reprogramming of my mind.

I was so determined that I was eager to do anything to turn my life around. My readiness to find out more like you was what gave me hope as well as the inspiration to change. One thing I learned a great deal about is the topic of mental programming and precisely how to use my ideas and even emotions to produce my truth. That is what this phase is about, and I think you will profit substantially from making use of some of the following methods

Imagination

The Power of Imagination is the most effective tool that people have been offered. It is the faculty of creativity. No other person in the world can imagine situations before they can occur (as for we understand it to be). Creative imagination provides us with the capacity to predict ourselves into the future as well as plan and prepare accordingly. But I assume vision is a lot more than merely a device for preparatory work. I believe perception is a literal maker of conditions and also events. I state this since I have knowingly created several opportunities for myself with my creative imagination, as well as I have seen several others make the same point.

What would look like 'lucky breaks' or 'coincidences' to the average individual are a routine incident in my life, and I am specific they are not mere coincidences? I could understand my thoughts as well as feelings to the point where things show up in my life by me only focusing intensely on them.

Everyone has this power, yet a lot of people are entirely not aware of it and utilise it to their detriment! Numerous people use their imagination to prepare for future occasions like something they are not looking forward to, for example. As opposed to thinking of things that excite and inspire them, they think of things that cause them to worry and get anxious about. The natural act of stressing over the possibility of failure increases the chance of failing because creativity is an imaginative faculty of the mind, not merely something neat to have fun. So now it's time to start utilising your imagination carefully.

When you understand these strategies I want to show you; you will undoubtedly be able to create anything in your life that you genuinely desire. A mind is a compelling tool, and it's time to begin using it responsibly. Even if you don't believe that you can develop situations with your mind, I would like you to act as if you can. Also, if it's not true whatsoever, it still serves you much better to take complete responsibility for your life

as well as not see yourself as a victim.
In my research study of successful
people, I have yet to find one that
doesn't believe that they create their
very own life with their mind. A lot of
the individuals who live terrific lives
do so extremely purposely. They
comprehend the power of their
thoughts and feelings, as well as they
use them sensibly to create the
experience they would prefer.

It's essential that you start to use
your mind intentionally as a device
for your self-improvement. You can
get to great heights, no issue where
you happen to be now, and I'm going
to show you exactly how. Your
imagination is your biggest asset.
With a little practice, you can start to
significantly change the program of

your life in whatever instructions you select. I'd like you to reserve an hour of your time to do the adhering to mental exercise. This strategy has changed my life and also many others, and I want you to experience the incredible advantages that it offers.

I will later address why we seem to have such negative thinking in the first place, later on in this book.

Beliefs Become Reality

The only distinction in between a person that is depressed and a person who is happy are their ideas and thoughts. An unfortunate individual will undoubtedly tend to believe constantly about all the adverse things in their life. They will undoubtedly take pleasant things and even attempt to place an unfavourable spin on them. Satisfied individuals often tend to see whatever in a much more favourable light. They make relatively unfavourable things and set a fun spin on them. You know, it's everything about understanding.

Two individuals can see the same circumstance and also see two completely different points. A single person could lose their job and see it as ruining their life, while another individual can lose a job and see it as a chance to locate to a far better one. There are no 'good or 'bad' situations; it's all about perception. It is an issue of belief. Occasionally experiencing these things is needed for development. For a lot of my life, I was an exceptionally negative individual. I would undoubtedly see out my life and think about all the important things I was disappointed with in the past. The world resembled a frightening and also aggressive place to be. I resided in constant worry.

Today, nonetheless, I see the world as a gorgeous place filled with a chance as well as exhilaration. I acknowledge my defects yet concentrate on my toughness. It took me years to shift from an unfavourable attitude to a favourable one, yet it made all the difference in my life. I went from seriously dispirited to very satisfied, and I can claim with self-confidence that it is just an issue of understanding and exactly how you accept that is the difference in between joy and also suffering. Let me provide you with a couple of devices as well as pointers that will undoubtedly aid you to end up being an exceptionally pleased individual. Several things have had the most significant influence on my understanding as well as the means by which I see the world.

Imagine Your Picture-Perfect Day

First, you will undoubtedly require a notebook or a few sheets of paper and a pen. You're going to be preparing out your optimal life on these sheets of paper, and they are most likely to aid you to make all your desires become a reality. This function marvels me still. It may be the most effective self-development technique I have ever uncovered. It is lovely to see your life ending up being precisely what you have visualised. Like I stated, the mind is a compelling tool.

Before you create anything, I want you to take a couple of minutes to envision your optimal life as clearly as possible. If you were living your wildest desires and also had no limitations whatsoever, what would your life look like? Currently, think of you having to live a particular day over once more for the remainder of your life.

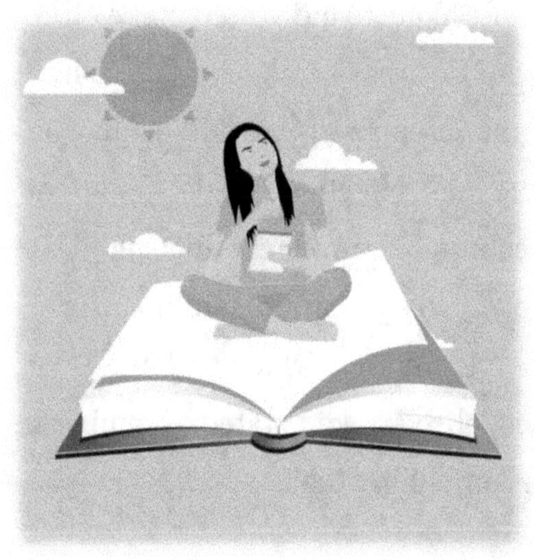

- *What would you want to do on that specific day?*
- *Who would you most certainly want to see?*
- *What would you spend your time on or what would you be doing?*
- *What car would you drive?*
- *Where would you be living?*

Think in as much information as feasible as well as attempt to picture yourself living this great life. Invest some time on this until you generate a clear psychological image in your mind. You are currently well on your way to greater things, yet the next action is most crucial.

Now that you have a clear image in the mind of your most excellent day, you will need to write down the description of it in excessive detail. This is your future you are intending, so do not be afraid to invest time in this exercise. It does not a matter in any way if you don't believe in your capacity to live your desires right now. However, it is essential that you do this writing exercise. Jot down exactly what you would do on your perfect day from the time you rise, until the moment you go to bed.

- *What would you eat for the morning meal?*
- *That would indeed you consume it with?*
- *What would your home be like?*
- *What would you chat to someone about?*
- *What would you see when you looked out your window?*
- *What kind of work would you do?*
- *What would your good friends be like?*
- *What sounds, smells, preferences, and views would you wish to experience?*

There are no limits to this exercise. The more detailed you get, the more reliable it will be and the quicker you will bring these things into your life. You could get as particular regarding state the colour of your room tiles or the shape of your sofa or bedroom perhaps the view out of the window. Invest a significant amount of time on this and fill it up with as many sheets of paper as you can. You will indeed thank me later.

Why is this workout so powerful? It pertains to the reticular turning on of a network system in the brain. This component of the brain functions as a filtering system and causes you to acknowledge just the things that are most straightened with your thinking.

You've most likely had the experience of purchasing a new

vehicle, and then instantly you start discovering the very same car almost everywhere you go. This is you turning on the system in action. It removes what's not crucial and focuses your interest on the essential things appropriate at the time.

With this composing exercise, you are permanently configuring your mind to discover things in your setting that assist you to reach your goals. The suggestion behind it is that if you remain to visualise and assume regarding your proper life, you will slowly yet undoubtedly start to recognise as well as attract things into your life and the assistance to get you closer to your objectives. You will undoubtedly begin to meet people and discover your conditions falling perfectly in line with your goals.

Ideas will undoubtedly start to fall right into place perfectly without you needing to do anything more than visualise what you desire. The sensation is somewhat mystical and can't be fully clarified, but it seems to work every time. If you grasp the rule of the law of attraction, then this ought to mean something to you. Otherwise, do not stress, because all you require to do is to start composing this workout and to see it at work, and you will end up being a follower.

As I have already said, you should visualise what you want. That is the reason why it is needed for you to draw up your ideal life in extreme detail. The in-depth description allows your mind to form a powerful image. The image must stimulate a specific emotion within you. The more descriptive you get, the more favourable feeling you will undoubtedly feel.

The description of your ideal day should make you feel delighted. If it doesn't, after that you ought to use more detail or find or think of a more explicit photo in your mind. This can be fun for you to do. Take a look at a few magazines to find your ideal image to start with and describe it instead for now, until you can imagine your image. Treat it as an amusing imagining workout. Once you have jotted down the complete summary of your ideal day, you ought to read it daily for at the very least, a month. Also, get involved in the habit of imagining your perfect day whenever you get the possibility.

Make it part of behaviour to continually believe in it regarding your proper life. The more you do this, the faster your life will undoubtedly change. The new favourable emotions you can produce within you when thinking about your most excellent life, the extra efficient the visualisation workout will be and the quicker you will discover significant modifications taking place.

Strong emotion mixed with thought is a potent combination indeed. Get efficient daydreaming about the life of your desire. This will frequently have an immediate impact on your mood. You will feel happier and be much more confident, particularly when you can instruct yourself that all your dreams can undoubtedly become a reality.

Do not stress regarding any action steps. Just imagine what you desire as well as produce positive feelings to the most effective of your ability and miracles will inevitably start to happen. Have belief and understand what this holds. Your dreams aren't as far away from as you would believe.

Reprogram Your Brain From Depression

There is a reasonable bit of work to be done isn't there? It will take time and repetition. But how do you get your brain to get rid of negative beliefs that have been ingrained in your mind for such a long time? The answer could be with 15 minutes of manifestation where all else has failed. You can use your brain to manifest and reprogram your mind.

Let me tell you a story, about a man who used to be poor and homeless; he had a poor mindset and learning new things never worked for him. He was riddled with negative old beliefs and thoughts as if his mind needed upgrading of software because it had

a hypothetical virus of wrong beliefs.
I am using a metaphor to describe
his incorrect thinking patterns here.

This person experienced the
following:

- *Financial money issues*
- *endless stress.*
- *Suffered from depression, anxiety and constant fear.*
- *He experienced little happiness.*
- *Suffered from addictions.*
- *Experienced grief.*
- *Was feeling powerless.*
- *Diagnosed with terminal brain and bone cancer at nine years of old.*

Nevertheless, he somehow transformed his life from the inside out!

You see, these days there are too many gurus around teaching you the wrong things. Most teach you that there is the only way to overcome this or that, but in my opinion, there are several routes that you can take and it what helps and suits you that matters! Everyone is different.

- What you focus on and pay attention to, creates your reality.
- We all have a story.
- Over time people develop limiting beliefs.
- This is the cause of your judgement and consequences follow.
- Your brain's editor defines and limits you with 'what if's.'
- Reprogram the editor for unlimited abundance today.

Reprogram the 'Editor' or your subconscious mind, and perhaps you can forget self help-books for good.

Imagine if you could update the Editor's software in your brain, to establish new neural connections in the brain.

Have you heard of Hemispheric Synchronisation? It means that both sides of the brain can work together. Rewrite your subconscious mind from limiting beliefs is like a miracle; you can focus and see clearly after that and therefore, you can manifest whatever you desire in life.

Similarly, with NLP and hypnosis, these work in the same way but over time; eventual brain rewiring to decode reality, so that you can focus on what you want and transform your life.

Ever heard of Quantum physics Wave and Particle (which is the reality, and the now). Here is a fact – when focusing, the observer collapses the wave into the particle.

So in the same way, your attention to something is what manifests your reality. This means that the wave and not declarations and affirmations alone, change your life. So when you want to change your current circumstances with what you want, some you find that your attention won't let you.

According to this brain science technique; this is the reason why the 15-Minute Manifestation works. Create any picture you want in your life. Click or type and search this link below to find out how to edit the editor: <u>CLICK HERE</u> or

go to https://maximiseyoursuccessonline.com/overcome depression

This technique could save you time doing it all yourself and money should you decide to go and see for example a counsellor of some kind.

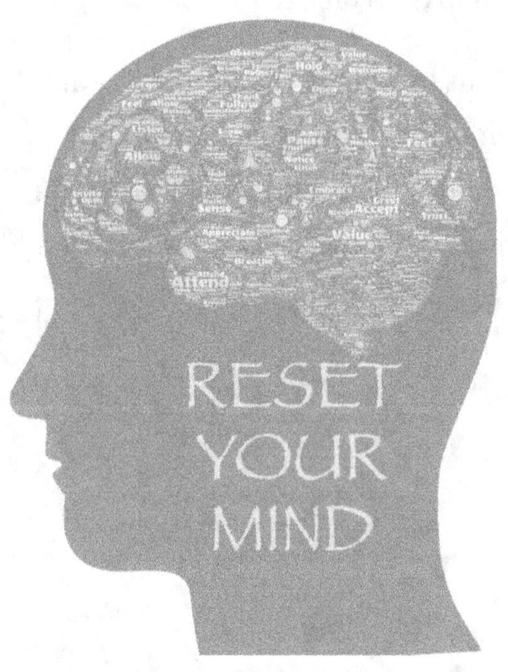

RESET
YOUR
MIND

<u>**What is 15 Minute Manifestation?**</u>

The 15 Minute Manifestation is a program that takes you just 15 minutes a day. The audio tracks are created using hemispheric-synchronisation technology audio that speaks directly to your subconscious mind, to help you eliminate negative thoughts and limiting beliefs. It's blended with a very high-quality, relaxing real nature sounds such as pouring rain, ocean waves, streambeds and wind. It is a truly unique and immersive listening experience. What's more, you can take it with you anywhere you go or listen to it while you're in

your bedroom or relaxing in the bath or the garden, in nature itself.

No learning is involved, and you can listen to the audio for 15 minutes a day, for 21 Days, which how long it takes for your brain to rewire itself.

Just imagine hearing real soothing "nature sounds" of theta frequencies and along with guided meditation scripts, that speaks to your subconscious mind. It repairs your mind to its normal state, back to when you were born. For example, abundance is all there is with no negative thoughts or scarcity thinking beliefs.

All the adverse circumstances and thoughts will soon get replaced, to what you want in life right now. It will lift your brain out of the misery and depression that overshadows you. You have nothing to lose and everything to gain from listening to this audio sound.

Right now, it comes with a FREE brainwave, *Deep Sleep Now* audio track with delta frequencies, reprogramming and guided meditation, for a short time only.

Transform your underlying mind conditioning. Your natural state of mind is abundance, not negative thinking patterns. You can download the program immediately today.

The method as tangible results; it has been proven to be the coolest and fastest to overcome depression or anything troubling you, and claiming your life back. People have asked if they can get the same results in other ways, yes but, most other disciplines do not know much about this method, to reprogram your brain. It would take you a lot longer and probably cost you much more money if you can afford it, to reprogram your thoughts.

Who can afford so much counselling or in some cases, take medication? Whereas, this method could help you if you are depressed about your work, money, illness, overeating or greaving for a loved one.

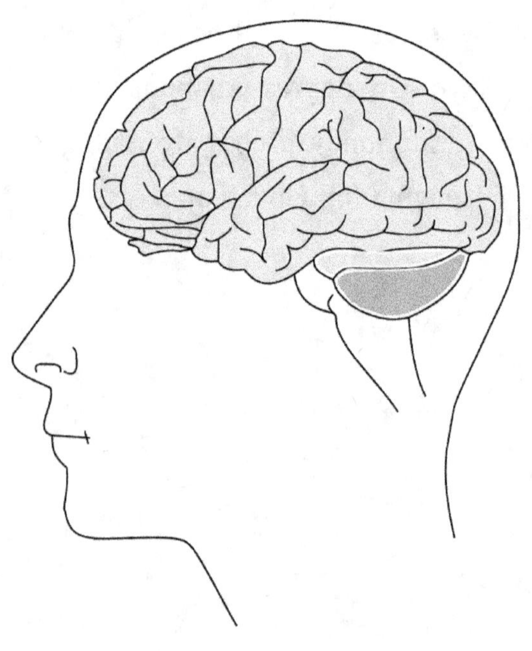

If you are depressed about, for example, food addiction and binge eating, you can try this too:

Go to

https://maximiseyoursuccessonline.com/overcome depression

or

CLICK HERE: <u>What is 15 Minute Manifestation?</u>

So far in this book, I touched on introspection, self-awareness and self-analysis, biology and nature predominantly, and how the brain needs to be rewired, re-conditioned or reprogrammed to think more positively. There are ways you can do this which is by journaling, positive affirmations or listening to audible affirmations to change old ways of thinking. Let's find out more about subconscious mind reprogramming.

The subconscious mind regulates the way we behave. We are mainly not aware of what takes place in our subconscious mind, yet it dawns in every element of our lives. We have been programmed and set considering that birth by our moms and dads, close friends, TV, songs, education and learning, and also whatever is in our atmosphere, whether that be good or bad.

Lots of people do not have a hint why they do the important things they do. That's because their activities arise from their subconscious mind. If you are presently dissatisfied with your life, you will need to deal with reprogramming your subconscious mind to make sure that you can obtain another outcome. The only way to knowingly configure your subconscious mind is with repetition. The repeat of specific declarations and also suggestions paired with feelings is a very efficient device for developing adjustment in your life. These positive declarations usually described as *affirmations*.

Affirmations have played a strong function consequently my life around, and also I think that every person must enter into the behaviour of using them each day. There are things you need to understand when utilising affirmations. Many individuals use them as well as see no outcomes because they are not using them appropriately. I'm most likely to instruct you an approach that will undoubtedly create you to see consequences exceptionally promptly.

Of all, it's vital to comprehend that words have very little power. The power originates from the suggestions that words stand for and also the feeling that they stimulate within you. It is essential to pick affirmations that make you feel excellent. A declaration such as, "I am rich" is much less effective than something like, "I am awakening to my real power, and also I will certainly utilise this power to live my desires as well as make a distinction worldwide." It will undoubtedly be different for every individual.

However, a basic guideline when creating effective affirmations is to utilise declarations that specify as well as empowering — usage of words that make you feel passionate and also determined. Your statements need to be effective adequate to provide you with the shivers around your body. That's when you understand they are functioning!

Some individuals do find affirmations overwhelming to utilise so it can be convenient to have them practising meditation.

Affirmations will subtly affect you, yet in time they will undoubtedly have a substantial effect. Bear in mind; your subconscious mind consists of years of demonstrations so it will undoubtedly take a considerable quantity of repeating for the affirmations to have a visible influence on your perspective and also understanding. Every word counts, however, so do not minimise the value of using affirmations. Utilise them daily, as well as you will undoubtedly see outcomes. It might take a couple of months and even a couple of years, yet that is necessary. The crucial point is that you are transforming well.

Integrate affirmations in every way feasible. Compose them, paying attention to them and then say them out loud while looking at yourself in the mirror Also, paste them throughout your home so you are compelled to take a look at them, or do anything that you can think about to guarantee you are constantly reminded to notice these words. The affirmations will surely reach your subconscious mind and have a direct impact on it. This is specially true when a soundtrack has binaural beats playing behind-the-scenes. Binaural regularities transform your brainwaves and also permit the subconscious mind to be set a lot more conveniently.

Examples of positive affirmations:

- *I enjoy challenges.*
- *I am a good listener.*

- *I am a fabulous daughter or son, mother, father.*
- *I'm creative in problem-solving.*
- *Better things are to come*
- *I can make a job stimulating and enjoyable.*
- *I can do this with ease.*

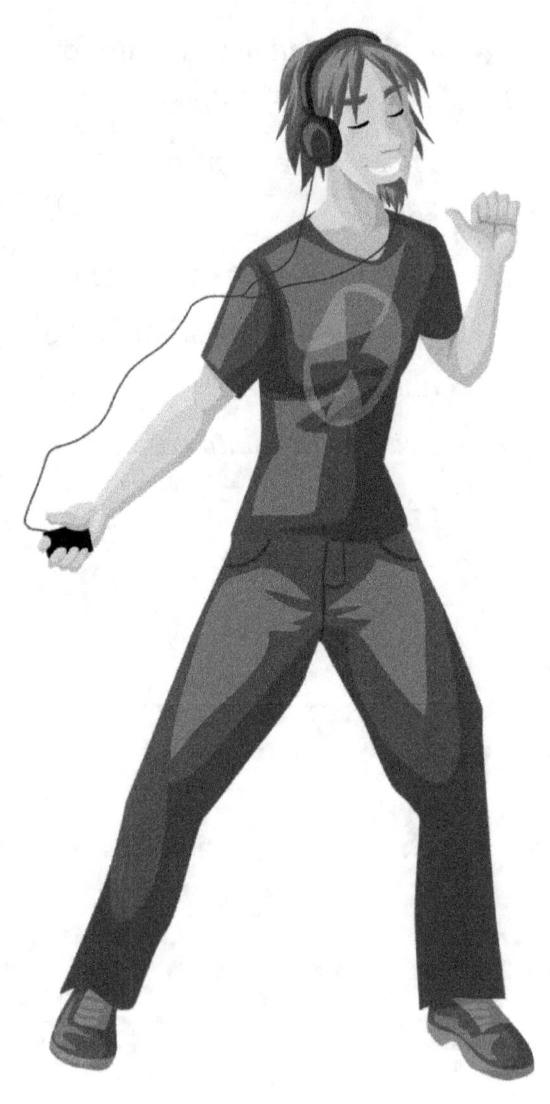

First of all, it's important to understand that words themselves have very little power. The power comes from the ideas that the words represent and the emotions that they evoke within you. Therefore, it is vital to choose affirmations that make you feel good. A statement such as, *"I am rich"* or *"wealthy"* is far less powerful than something like, *"I am starting to awaken my true power, and I will use this power to live out my dreams and make a difference in this world."* It is different for each person, but a general rule when coming up with effective affirmations is to use statements that are specific and empowering.

Use words that make you feel inspired and motivated. Your affirmations should be powerful enough to give you shivers all over your body. That's when you know they are working.

A lot of people find affirmations boring to use, and I mentioned that it could be beneficial to have them meditating.

However, affirmations will subtly impact you, but over time they will have a significant influence. Remember, your subconscious mind contains many years of programming so it will take a considerable amount of repetition for affirmations have a noticeable effect on your attitude and perception. Every word counts though, so don't downplay the importance of using positive affirmations or statements. Use them daily, and you will see results. It may take a few months or even a few years, but that is irrelevant. The important thing is that you will be changing for the better.

As I said, incorporate affirmations in every way possible. Write them often, listen to them over and over again, speak them while looking at yourself in the mirror, and paste them all over your house so you are forced to look at them, or do anything at all that you can think of to ensure you are bombarded with positive statements.

With an audio recording, you can listen to affirmations passively throughout the day. Even if you are

not paying attention to the words,
the affirmations will reach your
subconscious mind and have a direct
effect on the way you think. This is
especially true when the audio track
has binaural beats playing in the
background. Binaural frequencies
change your brainwaves and allow
the subconscious mind to be
programmed much more easily. They
are also relaxing and great to listen
to while doing another activity.

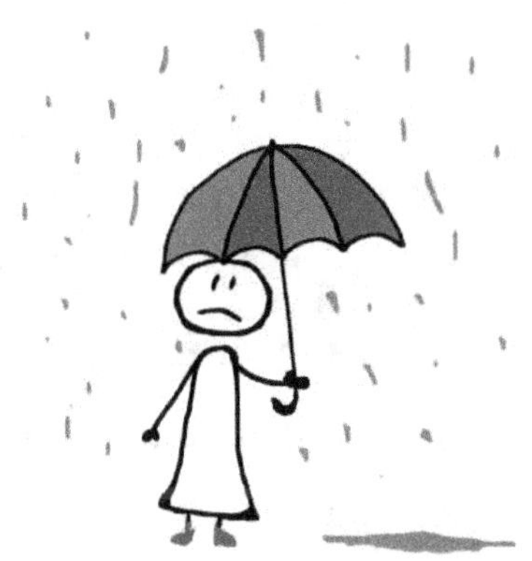

Find out more **<u>CLICK HERE</u>** or

Go to my website:

https://maximiseyoursuccessonline.
com/overcome depression

Feeling Depressed

Let me discuss a little more about feeling depressed or anxious. There are so many reasons why we can become depressed and anxious or sad. It is reasonable and appropriate to feel down, and even this is a sign of your unhappiness. Perhaps feeling of not having the ability to do anything regarding the scenario in your life or the sheer lack of control about circumstances; it may be a complication as well as deep worry concerning exactly how to behave, how to help yourself or someone else, for example, someone suffering from cancer or the possibility of losing somebody dear.

It is imperative to come to be experienced concerning the situation and to stay positive to make sure that it is not all doom and gloom. Even for example with a terminal illness, bereavement or grief, it is something to accept and to allow the feelings to enable us to focus and prepare you for more quality times with for example a particular person who could be dying.

It is necessary exploring precisely what your core beliefs, thoughts and also feelings are during this time that may show up as anxiety, and see if you can analyse or notice what those core beliefs/ thoughts/ feelings are showing you. They may expose things you might want to say to others or make small modifications in your life, perhaps do specific things you have never done before and so forth.

There are many ways you can deal with your emotions so try choosing something that will help you to channel and be more creative in your life.

Dealing With Stress and Anxiety Creatively

We are all creative beings. Our creative thinking has produced inventions that have enhanced the quality of human life; every one of which is the result of man's creativity. Suffice it to say; imagination generates artworks, which is such a large part of our everyday lives. We can see them in nearly everything, every room, as well as a wall around us. Artworks have been used as a visual means of communication and also expression going back to prehistoric times. Art mentions originality, an imaginative procedure, graphic materials, shades, appearances, spontaneity, danger, choices, and creativity.

But art is not just for the creative minds or the famous painters. Art is also a healthy and balanced way to share how we feel and manage our emotions. Art has been of central value to the healing methods of many societies throughout human history, and as time went on, through monitoring and study, an art-based treatment method created and called Art Therapy.

Art Therapy is a technique based on an understanding of human growth and psychological concepts. These are carried out in the complete range of models of evaluation and therapy. This can include educational, psychodynamic, cognitive, transpersonal and various other therapeutic means of fixing up emotional conflicts. Fostering self-awareness, developing social abilities, managing habits, resolving problems, reducing anxiety, helping truth orientation as well as boosting self-esteem.

The beginnings of contemporary art therapy can be traced to the very early 1900s when psychiatrists first speculated if there was a connection between artworks and also the diseases of clients. At the same time, art educators started to observe just how the free, as well as spontaneous artworks of youngsters, were a kind of personal narration which conveyed mentally as well as symbolically meaningful messages.

These two areas of interest eventually led to the emergence of the unique discipline of art therapy in the 1930s. Art specialists have come to be progressively organised, setting up graduate programs, expert organisations, and also journals.

A selection of artistic approaches is utilised in Art Therapy and divided into different specialist locations. Some creative methods that are made use of are music, dancing, psychodrama, movie, speech, leisure, and poetry as well as image treatment.

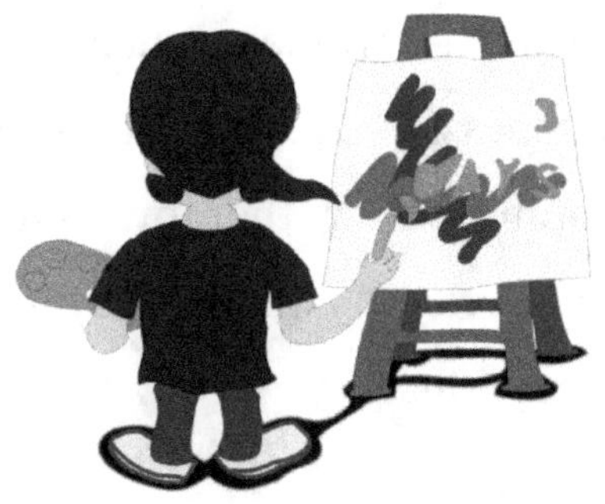

Drawing, or paint, help many people to integrate internal problems, launch deep emotions, as well as foster self-awareness, and personal development. Some psychological health and wellness service providers utilise art treatment as both a diagnostic tool as a means to assist and deal with problems such as anxiousness, abuse-related injury, or schizophrenia. Art therapy sessions are also given to jail inmates and HIV individuals.

Although there is reasonably little scientific evidence that verifies that it assists individuals with cancer, several health and wellness experts believe it may urge cancer patients to express their feelings, which can help them enhance their connection with others. It can additionally take their minds off from any discomfort and pain.

Art is discovered to be of the fantastic way most especially to a depressed person. Via art, they can find their temperament and express it healthily. In one research, art therapy was made use of with suicidal young adults, and the results revealed that it had positive effects as part of an overall therapy strategy.

An additional study released in the Journal of Pain and Symptom Management found that art treatment can minimise a broad spectrum of symptoms related to pain and stress or anxiety for example, in cancer patients. In the research study done at Northwestern Memorial Hospital, cancer clients reported significant decreases in eight of nine signs determined by the Edmonton Symptom Assessment Scale (ESAS), after investing an hour of dealing with art tasks of their choices.

Emotional disturbances such as anxiety overload, depression, or anxiousness are the result of losing touch with one's thoughts and ideas as well as feelings. One way to return back in touch with ideas and emotions is through the use of art. Art treatment provides a sense of success, pleasure, and also it is an individual expression for those interested in comfortable relaxation as well as self-discovery.

Let us look at other types of upset and emotions that leave us feeling sad and depressed which we can experience through life and the ways we can handle them, in the next section.

Coping with Emotional Pain

Emotional pain can often lead us to feel depressed and anxious. External circumstances can also leave us with emotional scars. We all go through some form of trauma in our life, whether it be losing a loved one, illness or divorce or any relationship breakup. Often these can be some of the most emotional and stressful experiences that can happen in anyone's life. Whatever the reason for your depression, it will leave a scar somewhere in your heart. It may take time, but getting through it is imaginable. There are creative things you can do to get over the

sadness, anxiety, and pain that you
felt because of it.

Acceptance

Most experts have said that the initial step to moving forward is acceptance. You need to accept the stark reality of any problem, that you no longer have that person in your life or you are no longer a part of the other person's life, and you are hurting emotionally.

Some people might tell you that they are just fine after a breakup even though they're still hurting inside. You should avoid doing this too! Rejecting the reality of your circumstances won't help you move on. The agony in your heart will remain until you deal with it appropriately.

Why is losing a loved one or breakups so agonising?

Romantic relationships are usually composed of beautiful moments and memories. Therefore, any loss of this magnitude with someone that was in your life will significantly affect your well-being. During the span of your relationship, you spend considerable time with him or her, so you're used to their presence. You'll surely miss them now that they have departed entirely from your life. A lot of things become uncertain and strange to you such as your usual routine, perhaps responsibilities, and your ties with people that are nearest to you and your partner.

Allow Yourself to Feel the Pain

You should know that it's okay to feel
confusion, fear, anger, resentment,
or sadness. To completely accept the
situation you're in, you need to allow
your feelings out and show it. Should
you need to cry, then go ahead and
cry your heart out. If you are a
private person, then do it in private,
no problem at all with that. But
surrender and allow yourself to
grieve for any loss caused by losing a
loved one or a breakup. By doing
this, you're going to move on by
letting go of these sad feelings. They
will never leave totally, but they
won't be so powerful and
overwhelming. You'll begin to feel
much lighter over time, believe that.

Resiliency

Resiliency is the capacity of a person to adjust to adverse events in their life quickly. It should help them balance themselves, their emotions, feelings, and decision making. After the hardships, they should still manage to maintain functioning on both a physical and psychological level.

People who are buoyant pay focus on giving more attention to their inner self-strength. This is why they can face life's problems. On the other hand, people who are not resilient are easily affected and influenced by stressful situations, often overwhelmed by problems, and can't balance their physical and psychological health at all.

Having resiliency does not necessarily mean that you won't face any difficulties, but it what it does is give you the courage to still find enjoyment and happiness after experiencing a divorce or losing a job.

Resilience

This kind of flexibility or elasticity is not an inborn trait, but you can cultivate it through experience. It depends on how you cope with the challenges that come your way.

Here are some steps on how you can build and develop resiliency in life:

1. be emotionally aware.

The reason why people are overwhelmed by problems is that they do not know their inner self and the capacity of their feelings. As you grow up, you must slowly learn more about yourself, your personality, and characteristics. In that way, you will know how to react to life's challenges.

To do that, you can start by writing in your diary or journal. Write down the events of the day. You should note down how you behaved and handled every situation. Evaluate yourself and indicate whether you did the right thing or you just let those situations affect you negatively.

2. Ask for supportive relationships.

Any individual would need other people in his life. Some people may handle themselves very well, and they are independent, but it does not mean that they won't need support from the people close to them.

If you are experiencing a low point in your life, then you need your friends and family who can help lighten up the load. They will give you much-needed advice and encouragement to help you cope up with the stress. In this way, you will not feel that you are alone. There are still people who are willing to help you.

The emotionally healthy people know how to ask for help so they won't

carry the entire burden by
themselves.

3. be positive.

Developing a positive attitude will
get you through most obstacles. It is
your way of encouraging and
strengthening yourself. Though
having social support is right, you
still need real strength coming from
your inner being.

If challenges come your way, tell
yourself, "Stay strong!" or "come on,
I can do this!" These are just simple
acts of courage, but if you believe
them, then they will be of great help
in overcoming the adverse situations.

4. Know how to control yourself.

If you develop the ability to control your responses to different events in your life, then you will be more resilient to difficulties. While the positive and negative occurrences in life cannot be controlled, you should know how to react better, and you are indeed in control of that! Remember, you always have a choice in every aspect of your life.

Do not be swayed by the difficult circumstances. Instead, face them and learn from them. It is your call if you will be either weaker or stronger after every adversity.

5. be optimistic.

It is about seeing things from the right perspective a bit like the old saying "through rose tinted specs". People will experience both sadness and happiness, but the optimistic ones are the people who know how to maximise the positive and minimise the negative things in life. Imagine viewing things with a pair of binoculars; you have the controls to focus and to adjust the view.

6. Do not give up hope.

If you are in a problematic situation, you will overcome it. There is always a light at the end of the tunnel, and sometimes things do happen for the greater good too. You need to know how to do whatever it is you need to do, but the main thing is not to give up, because you always have a way of defeating the obstacles. Besides, look around and see the people who are willing to support and help you.

Loving yourself is the first step to happiness. Without it, you can end up forgetting the value of taking care of yourself before anyone else. Invest in it by feeding your mind, body, and soul. You will be happy in doing so.

There are some tips and things you can do to give yourself some much-deserved love:

- *Listen to your feelings.*

- *Have compassion for yourself.*

- *Be open to changes about what your self-tells you.*

- *Surround yourself with loving people.*

- *Be kind to yourself and others.*

- *Manage your time and money wisely.*

- *Take care of your body and health.*

- *Look for a job that you love.*

- *Lead a balanced life.*

Emotional Healing

Let us take a look at emotional well-being and healing. When discussing health, most people think of physical fitness, sleep or rest. Whereas, others might think of nutrition and diet. These are all related to health but in the physical aspect. Fact is most people are not aware that the mental and emotional states are also crucial parts of the overall well-being of a person.

Both Mental and emotional health are different parts of who you are as a person. Most people think that they are the same, but here are the things that separate one from the other.

Mental health issues often necessitate cognitive thinking which includes critical skills such as long-term memory, processing speed, logic, reasoning, visual/perception and auditory processing, plus the capability to keep your focus and attention on particular tasks.

The brain is primarily involved in doing this because it processes every single bit of information that comes from your five senses. It takes care of how the body reacts and responds to external stimuli. Making choices and articulating opinions are also part of mental health.

It defined as your capacity to understand yourself and how sensitive you are to your psychological experiences. This also involves how you control your feelings and emotions, including dealing with and influencing other people. This includes how you're able to bounce back from the difficult situations in life, as I've mentioned earlier, and we know that not all of us have that kind of resilience. Every person would have a different response to emotional experiences. Younger people may have less understanding of life, so they can sometimes be overwhelmed by powerful emotions. While the older more senior people are often better able to control their feelings, they know how to handle difficulties much better.

So, in what way do they vary from each other?

Mental health helps a person process the information given or received by the brain for them to think and make the right decisions.

Emotional health refers to the ability of a person to express his feelings and emotions appropriately. Though they may involve different functions in maintaining your well-being, they are unable to be divided from each other. People often refer to them as:

- *the mind* (mental health)
- *the heart* (emotional health)

They need to be balanced so you that you develop the right attitude in life. When facing problems, you need to be able to analyse the situation first. Ask yourself, "*Why did this happen to me?*" or "*What are the mistakes that I made and what can I learn from it?*" After that, you can use your heart to make the right or appropriate responses to the problem. That is how they ought to work together.

Mental and emotional health needs to be monitored and looked after as much as your physical health. If you avoid it, you could end up experiencing psychological problems like depression, worry, anxiety, trauma, and often stress. Should you find you are not entirely able to process the information or control your emotions or feelings, it can end up cluttering your mind. This too is stressful and can often lead to other severe problems. And it can affect areas of your life, making it even more difficult for you to move on from any low moods, heartache or depression.

Having a healthy mental and emotional state will not guarantee happiness, however. As I've said before, every person encounters adversities and setbacks such as disappointments, loss of a loved one, breakups, and illnesses, as they go through life. They are inevitable I'm afraid. The only armament you have, for now, is your **inner strength**. I will give you an even higher power to learn about and lean on later in this book. But for now, happiness comes from your ability to listen to your emotions and feelings and in making the right responses to it.

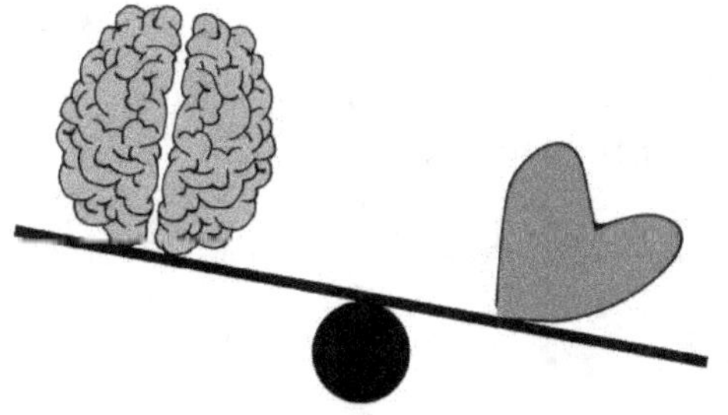

How will you know if you are mentally and emotionally healthy?

Emotional health can also refer to your knowledge about your feelings and behaviour. So if you are aware of the things going on within you and can handle things more sensibly and logically, then you can trust that you are reasonably psychologically healthy.

Here are other factors to help you identify if you are mentally and emotionally healthy:

1. You are self-aware of your thoughts and feelings.

2. You are relatively content with the life you have.

3. You are happy with what you already have.

4. You seem to have a positive attitude generally.

5. You have relatively high self-esteem and self-confidence.

6. You are prepared to learn new things and can adapt to most changes.

7. You balance work, relationships and time for yourself.

8. You have drive and determination, and you set goals for yourself in life.

9. You know what your main priorities are.

10. You generally get on with others and can accept your mistakes and learn from them.

11. You know how to find social support.

12. You can deal with problems and can get back up if necessary.

These are a few of them. Ask yourself if these are present in your life and if they aren't? Don't worry because these are precisely the things you can work on. At least for now, you know which ones you need to improve and develop when it comes to your

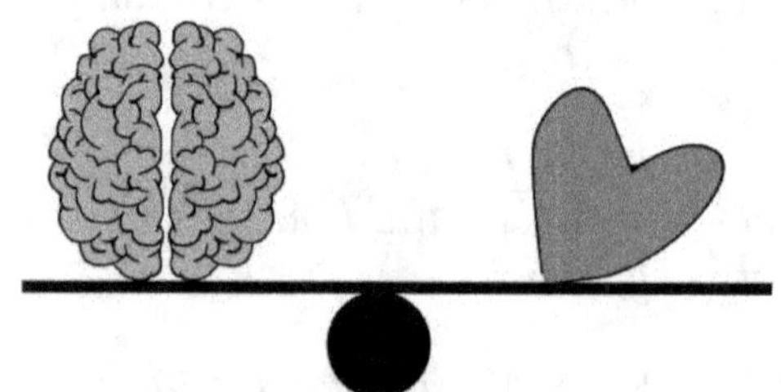

emotions and feelings.

Be Open to Supportive Relationships

You do most of the strategies and tips stated above. But, to achieve the best emotional condition, you would still need others to accompany you in your journey to "moving on" stage. People are not made to survive and live alone in this world. You ever heard the saying *"no man is an island?"* People are meant to connect and relate to others and to develop companionship.

Having someone who will listen to your struggles and suffering may help reduce the burden you are carrying. It is a way of releasing the heavy feelings and emotions that you keep bottled up.

It is not enough to find a friend; you must look for someone who can also become your mentor, supporter and adviser. They must be willing to understand your situation and listen to everything you'll say. If all else fails and no one can listen to you, then speak to a medical professional and seek help.

Friendship is a give and takes relationship. If your friend is always there for you, then you need to do the same for them at some point. Remember, these people will all experience setbacks in life too so make sure that when the time comes, you're as ready to listen and to be present for them.

The question is, "*How will you connect with other people?*" Here are some tips and strategies to consider:

1. Socialise outside Social Media.

It is true that you can make friends through social media, but it is not as effective as meeting the person face-to-face. Personal interaction includes the emotions, tone of voice, facial expressions and gestures. Relationships in the real world thankfully tend to be more successful. But do not go out and meet total strangers. If you do, make sure you tell someone and always meet them in a public place.

2. Go out and meet new people.

It is not good for your mental, emotional and even physical health to stay at home all the time. You need to interact and widen your network to gain more friends and knowledge about your environment. Choose to be with positive people, who are cheerful, and engaging. You need those kinds of people in your life, people you have something in common with often helps.

3. Join clubs, organisations, and other social groups.

When finding common ground, it often helps to join clubs, and you can turn acquaintances into like-minded friends. These social groups are your bridges to different kinds of people. This could be your chance to learn from them and share what you have learned too. You can create stronger relationships with fellow members, and it is an excellent opportunity to get to know people with the same interests as you.

4. Take time to help others.

Helping other people gives a sense of purpose and meaning in your life. It a remind us of sometimes being more fortunate than another person who is a great blessing. There are many people out there in the world who do not live a blessed life so you could make the time and have the heart to share your benefits with them. It is a great feeling to put a smile on someone's face or help them unexpectedly. I always maintain that somehow blessings do come back to you in some shape or form, for helping out someone in need. You can show your support by donations or money and also through volunteering to different organisations that cater to them. This can enable us to focus less on our own tiny or annoying problems sometimes.

Whatever is depressing you and it could be some things, here are some tips to help you to move on emotionally.

Love Yourself and Be Kind

The way you see and treat yourself will set a standard on how others would approach you. If you say bad things about yourself, it wouldn't be hard for other people to do the same. Remember, nobody can make you feel inferior unless you allow it, according to Eleanor Roosevelt. Therefore, love yourself, and then you can expect the people around you to be kind to you.

Learn to Forgive

Do not let the hate that you have for other people stay inside you. It can hinder your ability to love other people. Forgiveness is not about forgetting the bad things they did to you, but it is about letting go of the hatred and pain you experienced. It doesn't erase the past, but it will help heal the wounds it created in yourself.

Learn from both Good and Bad Situations

As I have mentioned before, every circumstance you encounter in your life is meant to teach you something. There will be good and bad times, but both of them can make you a better person. So, whatever happens to you, try to discern what it taught you. In that way, you will be a better person. And when a more significant challenge comes your way, you will be able to handle it better.

Stop Caring About What Other People Think or Say about You

They may say things about that are not appropriate for you. Negative thoughts that can make you feel awful about whom you are. Remember, if you know yourself and your truth, then whatever they say no longer matters. As long as you're confident, there's no need to worry about other people's opinion of you.

There will also be times when people would try to control your life. Stop thinking about them because you're the only one who knows what would be the best option for you is.

Let Go of the Past

The things, people, good and bad experiences in the past are done. You already learned what you could from them, so what you have to do now is to move forward. Do not let the past affect your present and future negatively.

Do not Fear Failures

Everyone is afraid of something. You may have a fear of failure or changes that may happen in your life. But the thing is, failing at some point in your life is normal. You wouldn't always succeed in the things you do. But, let it be a lesson for you, something you can use for your next task. The worst thing that failure and changes can affect you with is the fear of making another mistake. Never stop trying. A lot of successful people have failed a thousand times, but these didn't stop them from trying again.

Have No Regrets

There are things that you can never control in this life, so you must live your life the way you want. Give your best in everything you do. Learn from every mistake and failure. Never let other people control you. Just live your life to the fullest. And if you know that you did that, you can easily let go of your regrets.

Be Open to Change

Change is the only thing continuous in this world. Do not be content in staying within your comfort zone. There is much more to learn, and experience outside of it. Do not be afraid of the things you don't know

because that is when you can learn
and grow.

Appreciate the Simple Pleasures of Life

All the best things in this life are free. So, you don't have to worry about having not enough money because happiness depends on how you feel inside and not by the things you own. Learn to appreciate the small things that you have because they are the ones that can give you real pleasure in this life.

Do Not Cling to the Past

Your "past" is already a part of your life. During that time, you may have experienced hardships, failures, criticisms, and many more. It is okay to reflect at those moments of your life and learn from it. But, it isn't healthy to stay there, regretting what could have been. Learn to put the past behind you. Do not let it ruin your present and future decisions and goals. If you keep on lingering on the past, you cannot move forward.

Focus on the present moment, and plan for the future: one that highlights you, and not anyone else.

It is essential that you start doing things for yourself instead of depending on someone else's idea of what's right for you.

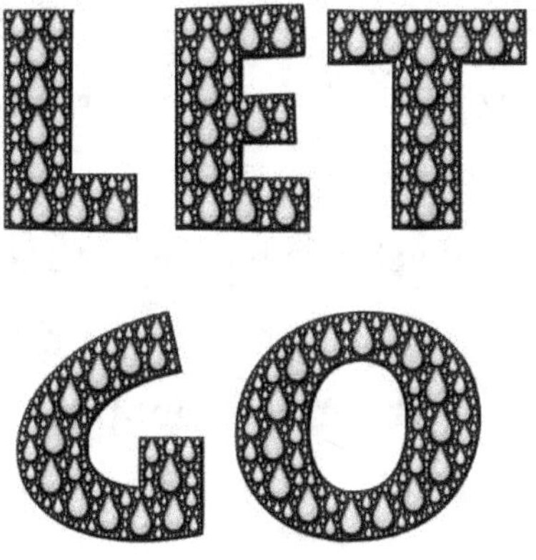

Sometimes, you might feel that something is not quite right or missing in your life. Have you asked yourself what it is? If not, ask yourself about the thing what makes you motivated to wake up in the morning and go about your daily tasks. Many people only exist, but they are not living. Your purpose in life is what keeps you going; it's what helps you achieve happiness and success. It pushes you in the right direction where you want to go in the future.

Coming from a bad breakup might take away your sense of purpose. So to help you get back in the right direction, follow these steps:

Know Yourself First

Before knowing your purpose in life, you have to know who you are: your personality, traits, likes, dislikes, dreams, and passions. In this way, you will have a clear picture of what you want to become in the future.

You can even get a journal where you can write about your thoughts and perspective about certain things. When you read it, you will gain a better understanding of yourself.

List down Everything You Want to Achieve

This is not only about material things, but also having a family or a good career. Jot down the thoughts about what you love to do, your dreams, interests and passion in life. These are the things that you enjoy doing the most and the things that make you happy, even if you're not paid to enjoy them.

Contribute to the Society

Always try and look beyond yourself because you are here to contribute what you can to the society. Determine the problems and needs of the community you are in and find out how you can offer a solution. Lend a helping hand when needed and try to work together with other people. Your interests and passions can make a difference to the people around you if used in the right way.

For example, you want to be a chef or restaurant manager someday. When the time comes, you can give back to the community by providing employment. You can hire people as waiters or cashiers in your restaurant. In your small way, you can help make a difference.

Look for Inspiration

There will always be people who have experienced the heartbreak you are feeling right now. These people have passed through their obstacles and hurdles before reaching where they are now. You can learn from their experience by asking for advice or help. If they are not within your reach, like world-known leaders or historical figures, read about their lives. There will always be material for you to absorb and take inspiration from.

Do Not Stay in Your Comfort Zone

Try to go out and see a bigger view of the world. There's so much to it that you might be missing out on because you are satisfied with staying at home. Explore the world! This way, you would be able to meet more people and experience things that can change you for the better. It is life's way of making you stronger and more confident in facing your fears. Take risks and know what you are capable of doing.

As you live outside your comfort zone, think of a better purpose for

your life — something that will help
you, your family and also other
people.

Determine Your Purpose

Now that you have examined and
evaluated yourself, it is time to figure
out your purpose. It might change in
the future, but what's important is
that you are slowly picking yourself
up and setting goals that depend only
on you. This should help you regain
power that you may have lost due to
heartbreak.

Stress and Anxiety No Need to Fret

Reflexes go off-centre, physical responses confirm to be inefficient, as well as habits patterns appear crooked with a mix of these bizarre incidents and also, by no uncertainty, you have anxiousness and stress; or a panic attack. Stress and anxiety are identified to be continual and typically emotional at times. Worries and fears that often tends to conflict with typical regular human behaviour or tasks.

Stress and anxiety, or its likely consequences, might cause problems but, research studies reveal it's treatable in nature as well as reacts to therapy well. Clinical developments, investigate treatments and an extensive range of responses that vary from anxiousness therapy to deal with stress.

Stress and anxiety therapies are done with medicines such as anti-anxiety medication, anti-depressants, and also beta-blockers. Anti-anxiety drugs are suggested for quick short-term alleviation versus anxiousness strikes as well as it is likewise made use of to interfere with anxiousness's extreme impacts.

These might appear to be the favourable payment of anxiousness therapies via drugs yet clinical individuals careful in way too much reliance on it. Anxiousness drugs can advertise substance abuse as well as, with this, enormous feasible unfavourable results are not needed to envision. They additionally suggest individuals take safety measure by consulting their routine medical professional or family practitioner. Medications can promote drug dependence.

Organic drug options and various other all-natural kinds of anxiety-curing practices encouraged as types of stress and anxiety therapy. If an individual is experiencing stress and anxiety issues, Cognitive Brain Therapy or CBT can undoubtedly assist an individual to recognise and get rid of the distressing experiences and thoughts that prevent the person from functioning and overcoming anxieties.

Dealing with stress and anxiety, nevertheless, is not that simple as it appears. It requires skills to get ahead of the problem the person had in the first place. The sensible and clinical based method recommendations the person follow the advice provided to assist with specific issues correctly, to work out anxiousness problem.

Likewise, family members of those handling stress and anxiety are urged to provide unrelenting assistance as well as the flowing quantity of persistence and understanding that this state of recuperation is essential for them. They are prolonging treatment and an initiative to allow them to understand that they are not the only person in this battle. This is essential to understand since one significant indication or display of stress and anxiety, is isolation.

Managing anxiety, as claimed by medical professionals, has no fail-safe or sure formula. It takes careful preparation as well as a continuous follow-up to be able to actually offer the very best assistance and also take care of individuals managing stress and anxiety.

With this, allow us to place in our minds that, stress and anxiety can be dealt with as well as it does react appropriately to therapies. Despite how severe worry may be, tell yourself, "Stress and anxiety? There is need requirement to fret."

Depression, Anxiety and Relationships

Depression and anxiety can be a lonesome ailment, and your relationships can often be an essential component of just how you manage your depression. You require friends for assistance. Not just fair-weather friends but good friends that can sustain you when you're down. If a close friend is likewise depressed or sad as you are then, it is not always a negative thing. You can comprehend each other at least and support each other on various bad days (but not if you're suffering at the very same time!).

Nevertheless, you need to be aware when choosing a partner or companion that your depression will undoubtedly have changed you as an individual. It is most likely that the person you are with each other when down will certainly not be the person you intend to be with when you are feeling much better. When you are depressed or anxious, you are a different individual. You might not also understand who you indeed are; however, your companion will undoubtedly be with the person you become at that time. Additionally, depression modifies the way you view things and consequently the way you see individuals; so your view of your companion will indeed not coincide with your opinion of them when you are much better!

I'm not stating that you should not begin a friendship or partnership connection when depressed. It could be the most useful thing for you to do. It might offer the security you require to begin resolving your troubles, and you might have the ability to talk with your partner regarding things you cannot review with anyone else.

Your companion might be the only individual you can unwind and relax with and begin to feel yourself once more. Problems might emerge that had not previously and would not have shown up if you weren't in a relationship perhaps. On the other hand, you might realise that you maintain the pretence of being the individual you believe you should certainly be. There is likewise the opportunity that the partnership might fall short before you being ready for a relationship - possibly because of your depression. This will undoubtedly make you even worse. In either case, the security of a relationship might provide you with the motivation to begin seeing things in different ways and the self-confidence to start looking for treatment therapy, if necessary.

Nevertheless, what I highly recommend if you do not begin a sexual relationship with somebody that is likewise depressed. I am not a physician, but there are two most likely results of this kind of connection. First of all, one of you will undoubtedly improve, and then you may part while the other may become worse.

If you are just close friends with a depressed individual, you can help each other, and if one improves, you can still help each other with your understanding and guidance. Nevertheless, if you remain in a partnership with a depressed individual and one of you improves, and then you broke up after that, the other individual will undoubtedly have endured the end of their partnership plus the loss of their friendship and help. Of course be good friends with various other depressed individuals, most of us require close friends when we're dispirited, but wait up until you have both recouped before you consider beginning a sexual relationship.

Depression can be a challenging condition, depending on the level of depression, to get rid of sometimes but it can be done. As soon as you have had it, there is always the chance of a re-occurrence. If you have recouped from your depression yet are still in a relationship with a person that is depressed too, it is tough to remain recouped. Likewise, you might find that you wish to leave the partnership but feel entrapped since you understand that the other individual will become worse. The anxiety of this might send you back right into depression and anxiety.

This is the second outcome in which case you will both stay depressed.

There are two likely results - the initial is that you could both improve and remain with each other. I think this is possible but highly unlikely. You could both be very different individuals when you are much better, with different views as well as character changes from when you initially met each other. You might desire different things. It would certainly be terrific if you both take care of and help each other with depression yet the typical tensions and stress of a partnership can make this not very likely.

The other result is that if you might improve, and you will remain with each other, but I still wonder if this is the least most likely to take place. If you recoup from anxiety or depression and manage to cope with somebody else that is depressed, then you are probably the least likely actually to be happy. You might still bear in mind the feelings and understand them, yet there might be a component of if you could survive it then they must have the ability too. All of us recognise that to be unreasonable behaviour when you have overcome depression which is the feeling that you cannot put up with others lame attempts to get better sometimes. Overcomers can often become dreadful critics, and sometimes they can be highly empathetic too.

Keep in mind that a lasting relationship is not always a bad thing when you are down and depressed yet, please think of the repercussions of being in a sexual relationship with each other if both of you are depressed. Attempt to assist each other as well as be there for each other yet maintain an adequate range of distance between you to ensure that you help each other and not bring each other down. To put it just, do not plunge into any relationships when you are feeling depressed but remain pals and do not attempt to move in together, at the very least, not until you understand who you are first.

Choose to Feel Better

Remember that you are in control of yourself. Attempt to make the rest of life impressive as well as cherish what time you have; giving thanks for every single day ahead which most of us we often take for granted. Instead of dread of a particular time or day, keep trying to enjoy making sure that you can reflect and look back on life and think, "*That was a fantastic time, or I had a great time doing those things.*"

You might become aware as quickly as possible, of the genuine, real importance of life, as well as its primary essence for you. You are then able to see the wood from the trees and be able to filter out all individuals as well as things in your life that do not matter. Conserve as much time so you can be on your own, with family members or special people in your life and try to invest quality time with them. Life is short so do things that you never did before together.

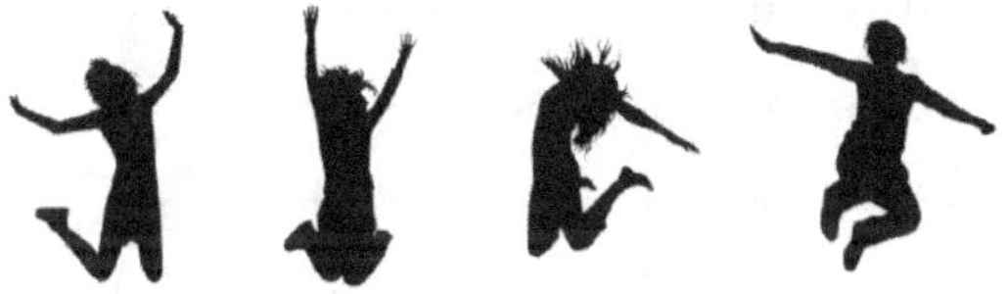

Easy and Quick Ways to Improve Your Self-worth

Self-worth is sometimes not easily attained because it takes a great deal of effort and also guts to encounter unfamiliar scenarios. You additionally require to work with your behaviour, instabilities, fears, and modifications daily to see improvements in you. Checking out a lot of write-ups and also blogs about getting self-confidence will certainly not aid you to acquire it; you additionally need to take action.

1. Have a rule

You can do this beyond meditation. Many people utilised rules when you encountered a difficult situation. You may have done this before automatically. Have you ever before given on your own a pep talk before a big occasion? Maybe a discussion that's essential to your work? There are those phrases that offer you strength and confidence to deal with the obstacles before you. It's always best to choose your mantra, yet in some instances, you can also make use: "I can do it!' or "I have prepared as well as practised for this, so there's no way I'm most likely to fall short." Keep in mind to say the words out loud or before a mirror.

This could make you look silly, yet it helps.

2. Speak to individuals near to you.

Self-confidence can also be achieved through the help of others, particularly those that are close to you. They know who you are, your toughness as well as weaknesses so you can trust them to provide you with honest compliments and comments. They can also offer encouragement which must reduce any tension as well as fret you might be harbouring.

3. Smile.

Smile when you do not feel like grinning. Then gradually, it will lift your state of mind. Frowning or having an unemotional face, can end

up aggravating the stress in your
body.

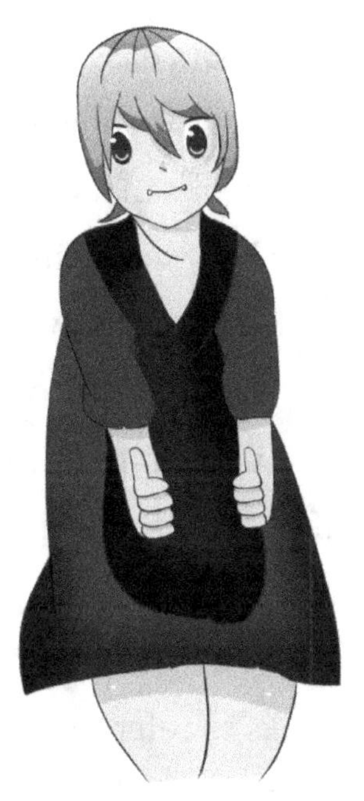

Be Open to New Ideas of Individuals You Wish To Be Like

There are simple and easy ways to accomplish every little thing you want. Discover books that can show you how to live how you want to live, and after that learn precisely what you can do. If you can start to see like a competent and delighted successful individual after that, you will positively turn into one all on your own. This is why it is necessary to have good books to refer to and examine the lives of individuals that are living their dreams and desires. If you are still depressed after that, your present ideas are not yet lined up with your objectives.

Just changing your perception will have an extensive effect on your life, which can be done relatively conveniently by learning more about the thoughts and ideas. This is not so challenging when you think about that a lot of the productive individuals of the world have created books or had publications blogged about them. Checking out these individuals will undoubtedly help you to become more like them. It is a widely known reality that all great leaders are our companions alongside our journey.

If you wish to achieve success and are delighted to learn more about self-education, take a look at several of the very best of my publications. These books can help you a lot if you

do not take pleasure in further self-
analysis; most likely require learning
more about other things. However,
you have the choice to listen to some
of my audiobooks (*see Books by This
Author*).

Checking out these publications will
undoubtedly assist you to move your
way of thinking to a much more
favourable one. I associate a lot of
my joy today to my routine of daily
analysis. When you review
motivating books, you embrace the
suggestions that guide you virtually
by osmosis. You will undoubtedly
start to think and believe in different
ways, and also as you do, you will
undoubtedly see adjustments taking
place in your life.

There is a law of attraction and an equilibrium that takes place; your exterior atmosphere (scenarios, individuals, events or an occasion) will certainly constantly match your inner setting (ideas as well as feelings). When you alter the means you believe, you adjust your whole life. It cannot be different.

You have been given some more tools to deal with depression and anxiety so take a look at a few more.

Steps to Avoid Depression

As we already know, there appear to be numerous people feeling depressed that we must take a look at the causes of anxiety in the first place. The elements that add to clinical depression are popular and well-researched, yet what creates it is not quite comprehended. Brand-new studies have uncovered several of the variables that add to the possibility of individuals establishing anxiety.

Anxiety

Tension takes the first place reward. It's true that any difficult atmosphere or circumstance can result in clinical depression. It can be anything such as social anxiety, obtaining a task, connection problems, fretting about money, staying up late, a way of life unmanageable, pressures of school and also getting excellent grades. Other occasions that could create depression are: death, change of work, relocating from one location to another; even the anxiety of the unknown can create depression. The listing is unlimited. While these occasions cannot be stayed clear of, we must develop a reliable tension dealing device to be able to grow also in demanding scenarios because they are never going to disappear. Stressful circumstances maintain altering.

Individuals that take drugs and alcohol are a lot more susceptible to anxiety. When these substances are made use of at a young age, they can affect a person's mind in unfavourable ways. These compounds help prepare the individual to feel good briefly, but most of the times, individuals come to be addicted.

Drugs launch dopamine in the pleasure facility of the mind. For instance: tasty food boosts dopamine release by about 50 per cent. Sex, on the other hand, doubles this number. However, medications can raise dopamine release anywhere from 4 to ten times. This unnatural high probably causes anxiety after the high vanishes. This compound is the surest way to fry mind wiring.

Medications make a person depressed more than it makes him satisfied. This impact will spiral downward till the person doing medicines will want more and more of the compound to damage the cycle of anxiety that follows each high therefore the dependency is birthed.

Not nearly enough sleep

Studies show that as much as 40 per cent of adults do not obtain the correct amount of rest each day and also among pupils, approximately 71 per cent suffer sleep disorders as well as the absence of sleep.

Rest is vital to a person's health and wellness. Throughout rest, the body repair services itself as well as reorganises thought. Lack of sleep contributes to an absence of comprehensibility in brain waves. This situation typically causes depression. Sleeping during the day and also staying up late also hinders the body's natural rhythms. This can result in a sense of hopelessness or despair.

Below are few means on just how to prevent depression.

Sleep is an integral part of stopping anxiety. Balance your life with adequate remainder as well as exercise every day. Many people need seven to 8 hours of sleep daily.

Keep some uniformity in your life. Organise your activities, so they can come with expected as well as average times. If you're weekly, every day or month-to-month regimen set, then your body has time to obtain utilised to the tasks. This will undoubtedly lead to a reduced possibility for clinical depression to embed in.

Don't push yourself beyond your limits. Keep tension in check and try to avoid stressors if you can. If this cannot be done, after that try to handle the stress factors in a way that decreases the damage it causes.

Sunshine, as well as exercise, can assist the brain to operate a greater degree. Make time to delight in the sun and try to remain active in the daylight when possible.

Avoid alcohol and also drugs. They may appear attractive, yet all they do is reason havoc in a person's life. Make at least one hot daily meal a concern. Excellent eating routines and health are essential when avoiding depression.

Have a good time each day. Nothing takes the lots off of anxiety like some tremendous fun time. Social activities such as conversation, linking to a support system sporting activities, as well as various other leisure activities can do wonders in the direction of healing a stressed out and restless mind.

Depression can be stayed clear of
and also dealt with, and it can be
enjoyable doing so. Follow the above
ideas for a brighter and better
disposition every day. You will
undoubtedly look and feel far better
for it.

However, sometimes depression and
anxiety can have slight advantages
too, read about this in the next
section.

Tips for Battling Depression and Moving On With Your Life

As you know by now, lots of people feel despair at some point in their lives. You might feel depressing over shedding your task, or a loved one died, and this is an entirely natural response to the problem. However, if the unhappiness does not disappear, then you might be dealing with depression. This section will offer you some pointers on anxiety, and how to combat it.

People experiencing severe anxiety or depression might take advantage of consuming foods rich in omega-3 fats or seeking fish oil supplements as part of their day-to-day diet. A research study has shown that omega-3 fatty acids play a significant brain function. Good natural fish resources for omega-3 fats consist of salmon, sardines, mackerel, and also tinned tuna. Omega 3 likewise plays a vital duty in heart wellness, so the benefits to your body are incredibly substantial without a doubt.

Do not increase the overload your mind and body are feeling by viewing a great deal of TV. There is excessive random turmoil occurring worldwide on the TV especially the news, or using computers and smartphones such that attempting to stabilise and balance your mind is almost impossible. Switch off the television and opt for a stroll, the garden or take a hot bath instead and relax. If you are outside, pay attention to the sounds of nature and attempt to disregard the disorder and confusion around you.

Consider therapy to treat your symptoms of depression if it feels severe. While many individuals don't want to do this, it is necessary to speak to somebody regarding the problems you are having. They can help you find other means of thinking of things and also assist you to develop a plan of action on how to tackle any depression effectively.

The difference between clinical depression and sadness or unhappiness resembles the difference between a water hosepipe and a dripping tap. If you feel you have been sad for no reason or continued to be depressed for a long time, there is a chance you could have clinical depression. Make sure to seek professional help.

Seek out motivational speakers when you feel down and depressed, or your inner voice seems expressively negative. Do not allow the voice a chance to bring you down and when you feel your inner guide start to be negative and harmful, as I mentioned earlier in this book, grab your journal or a recording of your favourite inspirational audio and let them be your inner guide for some time. It will fill your mind up with uplifting words as opposed to pessimism.

Again, self reflect, because reflection has been confirmed to be one of the most reliable means of managing anxiety signs. Reflection or thinking encourages distant observation of ideas, rather than the experience of ideas, and it can be very calming and give you the feeling that your worry has been alleviated from your shoulders.

If you suddenly start to feel depressed, take a close take a look at any medications that you are using. Some remedies or medications, even over the counter medicines, can have adverse effects. Altering the drug, or eliminating it when possible, could provide you with some alleviation. Review this with your medical professional, before any making any changes.

As specified at the beginning of this book, feeling unfortunate over the loss of a loved one is normal. If nevertheless, the sadness does not decrease later on then you might be dealing with clinical depression. Ideally, I hope this will help you to recognise anxiety or depression and how to manage it. If you feel you are suffering from anxiety or depression, never feel ashamed about asking for help.

Depression and Anxiety
Can Have Advantages

You might not see it yet; however, I can guarantee you will discover this someday soon. The contrast of depression and anxiety is essential for us to live the most effective lives feasible. We develop more as individuals when we conquer our battles, similar to a tree swaying with the resistance of the wind. Accept the conflicts and battles sometimes, and go along and bend with it; do not try to withstand it. Admit it like a boss and also try to understand that you will triumph. Your fight does not define you at all, but your capacity to conquer challenges does.

I've spoken to and researched lots of very successful individuals that appreciate their lives entirely, and have experienced severe anxiety and depression besides problems for long periods in their life. Individuals who cannot put up a fight can often never expand and grow either. Consider yourself incredibly honoured to be battling away, since you will overcome this and be far more durable once it's over. Each person can live happy lives. You might be challenged now, yet you will someday live wholly should you consider and use the techniques and suggestions I've provided in this book. You will undoubtedly go far, my friend. I count on you to do so.

Get out of life what you are worthy of and never allow yourself to opt for much less. Love being on your own. Advise yourself on a daily basis of exactly how wonderful you are. No person can tell you any different since you are the developer of your truth and destiny. It begins from within remember. Allow that light of yours to sparkle intensely to reveal to the world what you're indeed made from. For even more life-altering personal growth suggestions, check out my books and audiobooks on the back page.

But before you do, please read the next chapter.

What Therapy is best for Dealing with Depression

This part of the book is based on a mini research project that has been compiled for the purpose and aims to evaluate two or more approaches in the treatment of depression, critically.

Should you consider counselling or medication, then this section shows you some of the advantages and disadvantages of both approaches.

The first approach is Person-Centred Theory [PCT] and Clinical Approach. The complexities and processes of PCT are discussed and how PCT can work in this area. The objective is to explain the main differences between a scientific and humanistic approach towards depression. The researcher will define the biological and psychological depression giving a brief overview and evaluation of the methods including the advantages and disadvantages of tackling depression and other issues or limitations that may need to be considered in PCT. The 'person' will be referred to as the 'Client' or, 'Self'.

In psychology, there are various philosophies or, epistemologies that view humans from different angles [diagram A], in this case, depression.

DIAGRAM A

EXPERIENCES/
EMOTIONS,
CONSCIOUS
[UNCONSCIOUS]
MIND
Using PCT
Nurture
PHYSICAL [THE BRAIN]
the Clinical Approach
Nature

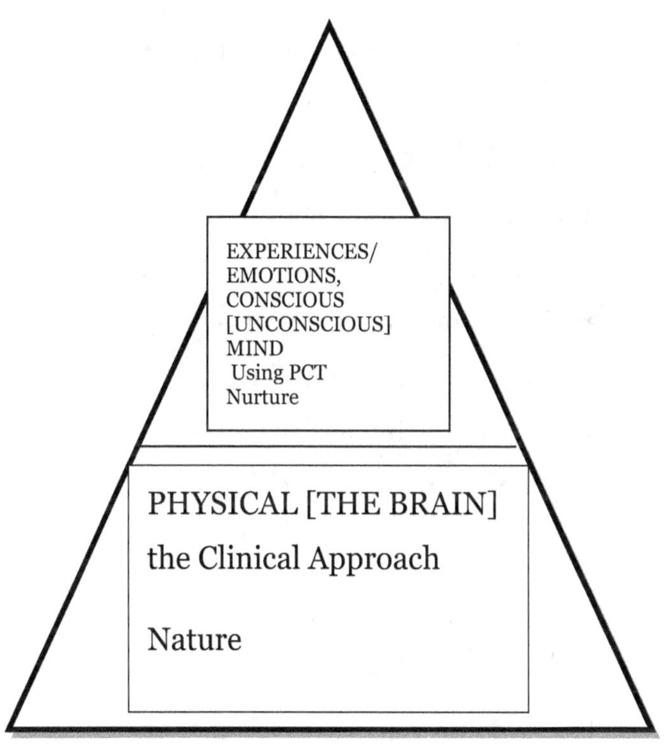

Some seek to objectify the person as a physical body or, a brain (nature), to diagnose and treat the person scientifically from the outside using quantitative methods. Alternatively, from the level of the Mind, a qualitative approach may be used to focus on the person and their subjective, personal experiences and environment (nurture). This is achieved by understanding and sensing what the person experiences and their view of the 'Self'.

Two Approaches

The two approaches are almost at opposite ends of the spectrum, i.e. natural science (nature) and humanistic psychology (nurture).

Known as the nature versus nurture controversy. Both seem to answer questions at different levels, but the former nature might explain the cause, effect and resolution in the treatment of depression, as opposed to nurture, the Person Centred method or PCT. In the latter, the therapist or counsellor provides core conditions to the client enabling personal growth and for the client to process their experiences and thoughts to help themselves.

Person Centred Theory (PCT)

PCT uses verbal communication to convey empathy and understanding to the person as a unique individual with feelings, emotions and experiences [*experiential psychology*]. The counsellor supports and facilitates growth and change by being genuine and providing the right environment or, core conditions for growth so that the client can feel safe. It is essential that unconditional positive regard and respect maintained at all times.

To begin with, PCT is a fundamental philosophy founded initially by Carl Rogers. The belief is that "the core of man's nature is essentially positive."

[*Rogers, 1961*]. Therefore, PCT is a way of *'being'*, and the person can express him or herself under specific growth-promoting conditions. When the philosophy is experienced and lived out, it enables the person to evolve and develop. The experience encourages growth and constructive change in others. There is a feeling of personal empowerment, and the individual can use this towards social transformation *"He is a trustworthy organism"* [Rogers 1977].

Therefore, the organismic-self requires stable development and growth, but there can be complexities during the process. To increase personal-empowerment, the person needs to feel uninhibited from societal *norms, rituals and*

rules by removing layers of values
and *beliefs* that are internalised and
introjected by the person from the
environment or culture that he or
she grew up within.

The core PCT conditions from the counsellor provide this i.e.

3 Core Conditions:

- *Congruence*
- *Unconditional positive regard*
- *Empathic understanding*

These conditions should be felt or perceived by the client before the climate for personal growth is possible. In the case of chronic depression, however, perception is effected at first.

Congruence

With *congruence*, the aim is for the counsellor to be genuine and open to feelings and attitudes within himself or herself.

Unconditional Positive Regard

Unconditional positive regard, the counsellor should try to experience acceptance and a warm, positive attitude towards the client; to accept the client in a whole non-conditional way even if the client behaves in ways which might conflict with the counsellor's values and beliefs. Therefore, without judgement, analysis and evaluations there should be an outgoing, positive feeling towards the client.

Empathic Understanding

Finally, with empathic understanding, this core PCT condition will fulfil when at each moment the counsellor senses feelings and personal meanings that the client is experiencing. Also, the counsellor can perceive from the inside and communicate his or her understanding successfully to the client.

In turn, during the therapeutic process, the client should gradually develop without having to worry about being judged or, condemned but instead, heard and more importantly, acknowledged and understood by the counsellor without the counsellor's opinion. In the counsellor perceiving and understanding the client's world with them, the client can begin to develop their self-agency by talking about experiences. This interaction enables the client to find their answer to possible conflicts and perceived problems. Thus, reaching an actualising tendency, i.e. fulfilment and realisation of their potential.

Regarding depression, for the benefit of the reader, it is necessary to define depression from both biological and psychological perspectives.

Life can often confront people with challenging circumstances; with going through stress, depression can be triggered by feelings of helplessness, powerlessness and repressed or bottled-up emotions. Other events, such as death, divorce, loss of a job or, physical problems from ill health like cancer can also become causes of depression.

The Biological Approach

Using a biological perspective, the centre of the brain has structures that regulate specific physical and emotional functions. These include appetite, sleep and sex drive. It also has pain and pleasure centres that work to control emotional expression and feelings.

When this part of the human brain functions normally, the person can eat, sleep and feels rested, they may even have a healthy sex drive. However, when a person is depressed, life circumstances occur and coping difficult. The person may feel highly overwhelmed by intense feelings or, exhaustion and loss in their ability to experience pleasure. Their threshold is lower than that of a non-depressed or less depressed person.

In chronic cases of clinical depression, this particular area of the brain malfunctions producing specific symptoms, i.e. loss of appetite, low sex drive, loss of sleep etc. This happens because of various structures of the brain start to shut down and need to be switched back on. To use an analogy:

If a TV socket is too far away in the distance for the plug, an extension cord is required, but in this case, two cables are necessary to reach the TV socket.

In the brain, electrical impulses activate via a network of nerve cells that are connected end-to-end like several extension cables — the electrical impulse travel along the brain cells separated by tiny gaps called '*synapse*'. The stimulation must chemically pass through the synapse, and tiny containers called vesicles, that are electrically activated by one (cell A) spilling out a neuro-chemical into the synapse [see diagram B]. The chemical messenger floats across the synapse and attaches to another (cell B).

Given enough chemical, cell B then activates the nerve cell, and another electrical impulse begins, to enable

the structures of the emotional brain
eventually.

With clinical depression, two problems occur:

- *Re-uptake*
- *Nerve cell malfunctioning*

Perhaps one cell re-absorbs the chemical, instead of it drifting across the synapse and nothing is left, therefore, to activate cell B. The second problem could be that cell B becomes insensitive and unable to activate after the chemical has passed from cell A, across the synapse towards it. Both issues are similar to the extension cords disconnecting towards the TV set.

The emotional brain [or TV set], then begins to shut down and symptoms of biological depression could emerge. If electrical impulses are weak or impaired then, for example, the person's perception of life and therefore their behaviour may be severely affected. Clinical treatment might be recommended such as anti-depressants medication or substances that are effective only to ease the intensity of the emotional pain and to restore the ability of pleasure. But this doesn't solve the person's perceived outer problems. However, it may not produce feelings of happiness whereas, tranquillisers which are chemically different, can often provide temporary relaxation or, euphoria.

DIAGRAM B

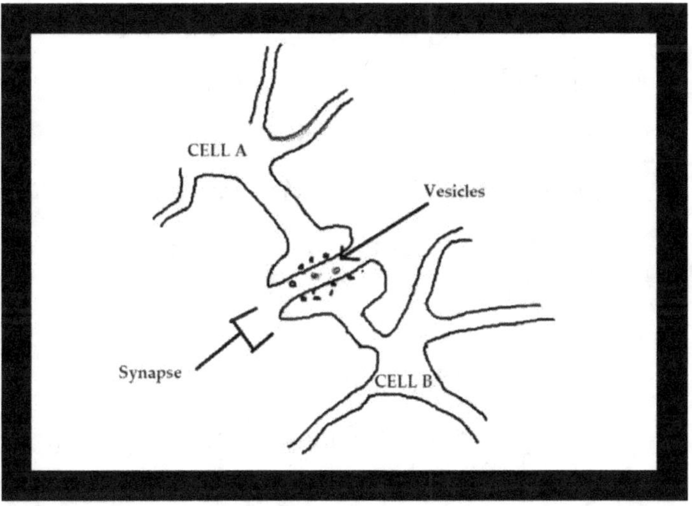

In contrast, psychological depression some experience as a lack of self-confidence or, self-worth perhaps due to traumatic circumstances described earlier or because there is a genetic chemical imbalance. The results being physical symptoms but also behavioural symptoms, i.e. inner emotional pain, denial, defensiveness, social withdrawal, isolation or fear and avoidance of contact.

Therefore, depending on the severity of depression, PCT may be more suitable for the person, i.e. to talk to a therapist and express their feelings, instead of taking anti-depressant tablets. With PCT the client may be able to get in touch with their emotions, by feeling completely accepted and supported with the PCT *core conditions*, from the counsellor. There may be scope for future change in the case of a depressive if their perception starts to shift. Perhaps longitudinal research studies may be required here, to test this area further.

It seems that both PC and the clinical approach try to support the client from different levels, one (clinical or nature approach) using general assumptions, searching for common factors, it places the person in a *'category'*, to treat with drugs.

Whereas, with PCT (nurture) there is a personal one-to-one *'relationship'* between client and counsellor. Quite possibly, medical treatment is not required if the client can process their experience and feelings with the help of a counsellor. Maybe both would have been necessary. PCT can enable the depressed person to work through issues and in time, gain personal empowerment and a sense of well being. However, there may be limitations in the PCT.

Firstly, the severity of depression may determine a limitation in the initial stages of the process in PCT because perception is affected, and therefore other complexities can arise for the client with an uneven playing field or disadvantage, that prevents them from going '*into the process*'. The physical brain might be affected by physical factors, e.g. hormones, post-natal depression or, Alzheimer's disease, and not necessarily situational life circumstances.

Carl Rogers believed that limitations of PCT could be *self-denial*; *distortion* or *denial* and lastly, *confusion and anxiety*. Nevertheless, PCT can try to look at the level of the problem using the *core conditions* and *seven stages of the process*, to gain insight. Whereas, the clinical approach, may provide very little support to the person's experiences and the concept of themselves while feeling depressed.

The advantages and disadvantages of PCT in comparison to clinical treatment are that PCT could be beneficial in raising self-awareness and reflection in the client processing past experiences and feelings. This, in turn, could shift brain chemistry and move them towards growth, change and freedom using the client's inner resources rather than the dependency on short or long-term medication.

The disadvantages to PCT might be that the client is too chronically depressed to perceive the therapeutic process initially, experiencing self-denial, distortion etc. The clinical approach might be a safer method to stabilise the person almost immediately, but as discussed earlier, medication will not address the person's feelings and experiences alone. Therefore, both treatments are necessary to first gauge the level of clinical therapy and or, further PCT, therapeutic processing.

Furthermore, in PCT counselling, consideration needs to be given to the interpretation and cross-cultural differences during the therapeutic process, and the person's concept of themselves and how their world is perceived and embedded within the process. Other variables might be a social class, religion; gender or, general outlook on life including language, jargon used by the client, e.g. when the counsellor paraphrases and reflects an understanding, it may be essential to clarify words and meaning for the client, and this could take time. There is also the question about who pays for counselling sessions.

It appears that both human diversity and universal commonalities are considered in both clinical psychology and humanistic psychology, as with PCT. Depending on the person's depressive state often linked to perception, self-worth etc., PCT may be appropriate. However, with illness or chronic depression, a more extended period of PCT processing may be necessary, but alternatively, a jump-start in medication might enable the person to perceive better before PCT therapy can begin.

For the benefit of transparency, more research over time is necessary for this area, i.e. to interview several participants and to compare results. The researcher in this project interviewed ten participants at had both clinical treatment and counselling. Participants confirmed most of the issues raised.

In undertaking multiple approaches [*known as triangulation*], assessing and then adjusting proportions of treatment or therapy, a broader holistic model applied to enable integration of the person successfully, not only from one level but from several levels, e.g. from the brain chemistry level to the psychological level and concept of 'Self'. Let us look at a third approach in the next section, one that is often overlooked.

Using Spirituality to Better Cope With Stress

The third approach I am going to touch upon here is the Spiritual Approach. As we know, the stress that individuals fight every day of their lives, not everyone has effectively handled it well. Tension is an everyday companion that is undesirable but which persists to be there from morning until you go off to sleep. It can make individuals miserable, flustered, short-tempered, and also extra prone to mental disorders and also various other clinical problems, as the body immune system get damaged over time. Unmanaged, it can cause anxiety and drive people to despair.

It is consequently not unusual that many numbers of people look for ways to be able to manage everyday stress and anxiety. Several of these are unfavourable like drug abuse, alcohol or food addiction. Some ways to soothe stress and anxiety, or hobbies, and then there is spirituality. Dealing with stress with spirituality is something that is unquestionably helpful as one ends up enlightened, and as a person's objective in life comes to be more explicit, there are noticeable changes.

Finding Meaning In a Person's Life

Unlike what lots of people think, the core worth of spirituality is not attached continuously to religion, though it can be. The dawning of awareness concerning self and the advancement of one's values leads a person typically to one's exploration of spirituality. This can be connected to religious beliefs because religion and faith are the most conventional devices in the direction of self-discovery. Embracing a philosophy like yoga that entails self-control with its Asana (postures) and also meditation using Pranayama (breathing) can lead one into the understanding of self. This can be important as this is the beginning of spirituality.

Exactly How Spirituality Relieves Stress

One of the most significant accomplishments that spirituality can provide to a follower is the exploration of one's sense of presence or reason of being. This makes an individual leave from materialism to relocate in the direction of the achievement of the better issues that define one's confidence and also spirituality. Thus, stress and anxiety become simply another unneeded thing that holds no value to the individual's life.

Stress and anxiety end up being an unnecessary concern that often tends to weigh down people's mind and also emotions. This affects the heartbeat, the stress of the blood, the functioning of several body organs and the weakening of the immune system.

Inner tranquillity is accomplished without effort regardless of seclusion as one develops the link with others and as one's old values are gotten rid of from every little thing. With chi or qi (favourable power), one becomes like a magnet that draws individuals and connections. This provides one the outlet to release, share or review with others their difficult troubles that effectively decrease the strength of emotions. As one unload fears, worries, anxiousness, pain, rage and also various other adverse feelings, the more that they become stronger psychologically and socially.

Spirituality also often tends to direct an individual toward a healthier lifestyle and even well-being. Quite often, difficult conditions at the workplace, in the house, and partnerships often tend to be exacerbated when one is destructive. As a result, a healthy and balanced way of life and also routines produced by spirituality aid a lot in decreasing and battling stress and anxiety. Quite fairly frankly, it is effortless for a healthy person to be satisfied, pleased, passionate, friendly, calm and socially interactive.

Spirituality has a significant role to play in any person's life. Managing anxiety via spirituality benefits a person in some huge favourable means. If you are struggling from stress as well as, have tried numerous ways to obtain it, but unsuccessfully, maybe it is good to attempt spirituality this time. So if you desire to achieve that higher feeling of enlightenment and handle daily stress in life, discover methods to exercise spirituality.

So far in this book we discussed:

- How we can do things ourselves like write journals and challenge our old believers. We need to write out positive affirmations. Staying positive and try out new things.

- We can use other means of
  changing our thoughts and
  updating our mind,
  visualisation techniques,
  listening to audios or bilingual
  beats to manifest better things
  in our lives.

- How we can deal with
  difficult, painful emotions
  after situations happen to us;
  forming relationships when
  depressed.

- I have explained Person
  Centred Therapy (PCT), and
  the difference s between
  counselling therapy and

treating clinical depression
with drugs.

- We have discussed depression
  in many different ways so far
  in this book.

- We have touched on
  spirituality but there is much
  more to spirituality, and in
  finding true happiness and
  joy, so let us read on.

The Reason You Were Born

Life, why were we born? Where do we come from? Were we put here by accident or is there a purpose on why we were put on this earth? It may surprise you what that purpose is.

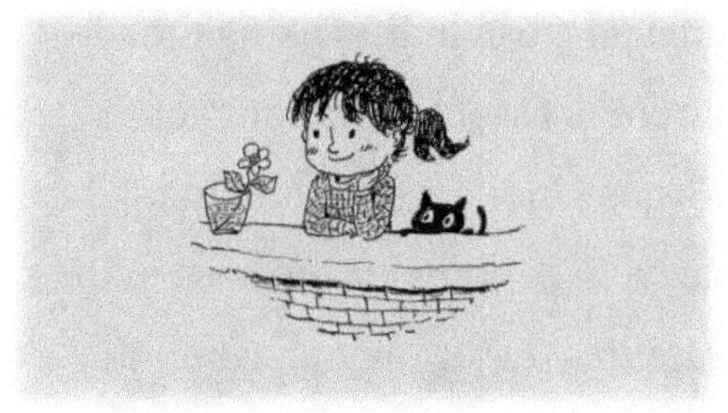

Happiness is the key to life. Many seek happiness through obtaining money, friends, personal achievement, family, but it's not your real purpose. Many people seek happiness or claim to be happy with man-made happiness but never really reach a stage of total fulfilment and happiness. There is a purpose far more significant than man-made happiness. Being a great employee is not your real purpose in life, finding the perfect person to marry is not your purpose in life, being the ideal parent is essential but not your purpose in life, going out and partying is not your purpose in life, watching TV or playing computer games. This is not why you were created. You can see how we have been brainwashed and manipulated so easily and subliminally by these external man-made things. Could this not be the reason why we often find ourselves sad and depressed? Could it be that our negative thinking stems from the horrific conditioning we have had since birth!

We're continually reminded of what we don't have, feeling inadequate, worried and lost, primarily through the media.

Is there any wonder we feel burnt out? Besides all of this, you have so much to do anyway. People have got their phones going off all the time, and then there are emails or text messages to reply to. Everyone is exhausted and need constant breaks, but somehow, you never seem to get that restful time to have off? What about the numerous spiritual practices around these days, telling us to slow down. People soon realise that a new outfit of a big night out isn't going to help either, not in the long term. People are becoming more aware of their wasted energy. Yes, we can talk to a therapist or perhaps you need somewhere to chill out, to relax and let go.

Then there are crystal healing, floatation tanks, Indian head massage, reiki or tarot. Everyone is told to tap into their intuition or to activate their third eye! Find out what the future holds and what your purpose in life is.

So, how do we find our purpose? We were created with one, and that purpose came from a much more significant, higher power. Therefore, finding true happiness on your own will often lead to failure and unhappiness.

In life we can choose many things all on our own, like our career, our friends, the restaurants we eat in etc. but when it comes to our purpose in life, there is one greater purpose for our lives. In the Bible *1 Timothy chapter 2, verse: 5* is the key to finding your true meaning in life, which is Jesus Christ.

Jesus was crucified and died on the cross at Calvary so that you can obtain eternal salvation and also can live the life that our heavenly father had planned for us all along. The book of *John chapter 14 in verse 6,* Jesus says he is the only way; the truth, the life and no one can come to God the father, except through Jesus.

When you don't accept Jesus Christ, you are working under your ideas and plans to achieve happiness which leads to emptiness, and something is missing. That something is the Holy Spirit within you.

Reach your God-given purpose in life. Establish this by book of *Romans chapter 8, verse 28*; all things work together for good for those who love God.

For example, you might be good at creating or playing music, and you might feel that it is your real purpose in life, but this may not be so. Your goal see *1 Corinthians book chapter*

10 verse 31, says to do all to the glory of God, not yourself but to please him and be in fellowship with him throughout your entire walk in life; he wants you to trust in him fully and to believe on him.

All things were created for God and by him see *Colossians chapter 1 verse 6*. So we already know from this Bible passage that we were created as unique and special individuals, to bring about God's Will in our life. We are already special in his eyes and loved very much by him.

In the book of *Psalms no. 139 verses 13-16*, you will read that he created you before you were in your mother's womb. We are his children, and each one of this world has nothing for us. The devil wants us to seek material things in this fallen world.

By accepting Jesus, *Philippians 4 verse 19,* Paul writes that God shall supply all your needs when you accept him into your life, you will indeed be genuinely blessed, happy and know your real purpose in life. Be part of Jesus' legacy and not the one you are trying to seek for yourself on your own. We have all fallen short of the glory of God. Jesus died to remove all our sins. Ask and welcome Jesus to come into your life, to be part of your life, and he will take over and lead you towards your real purpose in life which is to glorify him, and you will be truly blessed.

You have seen many tools you can use to help yourself in the previous chapters of this book. From: Do It Yourself to journaling; listening to positive affirmations and mindfulness. You found out more about dealing with painful emotions, daily health and fitness routine and listening to more audiobooks. I discussed the advantages and disadvantages of counselling and drug medication and then a third approach, spiritualism. You can do most of these but what next? Read on.

(Quotes from the King James Bible)

Spiritual Emptiness

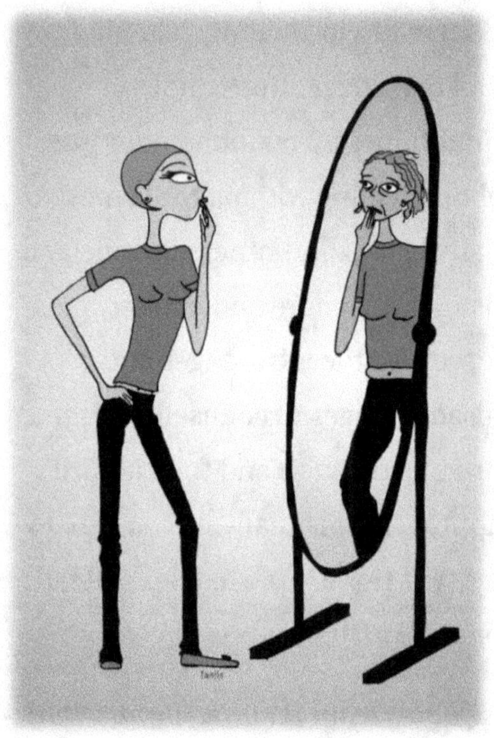

We often feel depressed for example,
just after Christmas and often into

the New Year. Why is that? The holidays and the parties are over. You didn't do anything special? Do you have too many worries and troubles? It can be a predominantly lonely time for people who have lost their dearest loved ones or have no family at all. Or perhaps you have thoughts about new beginnings and New Year resolutions, but can only see a bleak future instead with no light at the end of the tunnel?

With yet another Christmas been and gone, our thoughts should have naturally turned to the birth of Jesus. But somehow this world is far too busy with trivial matters instead. And more and more people are becoming disheartened with their lives. As I said earlier, at the beginning of this book, there are so many things going on — lawlessness, disasters, famines, earthquakes, wars and rumours of wars, floods. Unless you are a Reality TV celebrity, this world is somehow geared to make you feel inadequate, fed-up, empty, stressed, unhappy, lonely or sad and depressed. Have you experienced some or the majority of these things? It's why you may be reading this book!

I have provided you with suggestions earlier to tackle the brain your feelings and thoughts, and from the previous chapter, let us continue deeper towards the spiritual side of things, and I don't mean the watered-down New Age spiritualism or, paganism here. Some people might disagree but please first hear me out. I am not a preacher, but I am talking about the real one true meaning of happiness and promises with the one true living God.

As I said in the previously, Jesus Christ is our one right path to happiness. Here's the thing, so many people consider Jesus to be an instructor, teacher, a healer, and they would undoubtedly be right. The Bible, which is a supernatural, living and prophetic historical book, tells us that God guaranteed King David in ancient times, that there would be a son who would control Israel forever, in the future. That child is Jesus Christ. God never breaks his promises, and this had been fulfilled.

We typically forget that Jesus can declare the title *"King of the Jews"*. When Jesus was born, the three wise men asked Herod *"Where is he that is born King of the Jews?"* No one laughed, for the Jewish clergymen knew from the scriptures that one day a special person, a unique king would be born in Bethlehem. (*Micah chapter 5: verses 2, 4*).

We understand in hindsight that the last time Jesus as on this planet it was not God's will for Jesus to become the King of Israel way back then. But instead, The Gospel needed to be taught and preached to the whole world first, as it currently has been, to save everyone's souls. That does not mean Jesus will not be king over Israel though. He is King and will be King during his second coming (*the Second Advent*), sometime in the not so distant future.

The Bible informs us that when Jesus returns, his claim to the throne of David will indeed not resemble the kings that we see in the world today – Jesus will have the authority and also the power to claim his throne and the whole world.

The Bible offers us hope and a beautiful world, as it should have been before Adam and Eve broke God's covenant, by eating the apple from the tree of knowledge. The world will certainly not always be depressing that it is currently in – the physical violence, the corruption

and the wicked ways of the people
that we see today.

You only have to hear on the news to
see the terrible things going on
around the world today, and this all
falls in line with biblical prophecy.
The good news is that Jesus already
gained victory over Satan when he
shed his precious blood, and he died
on the cross, to save us; he was
buried and rose again on the third
day, ascending to heaven. These are
exciting times because he will return
soon before the seven-year
tribulation which you do not want to
be part of at all. So if you feel down
and depressed don't give up and read
the bible, please.

The Bible is the best self-help book
you could ever read, and it instructs

us that we can have that beautiful hope and joy in ourselves, which we will undoubtedly get and the chance to help Christ when he returns. However, we first need to do something regarding it right now. We have to recognise that Jesus is the son of the living God. Jesus had shed his precious blood, and he died on the cross for all our sins and rose again on the third day. He is now seated at the right hand of God, but he will be coming back soon to save us all soon. It means more than being baptised in the name of Christ if we are to live forever with Jesus and also with our deceased loved ones and new friends in all eternity. How wonderful and exciting is that?

This is what the apostle Paul stated when he explained what he was anticipating:

"Finally, there is laid up for me the crown of righteousness, which the Lord, the righteous Judge, will give to me on that Day, and not to me only, but also to all those who have loved his appearing." (2 Timothy 4:8).

(Quotes from the New King James Bible)

So, think of the birth of Jesus around Christmas, but additionally, consider the reasons that he was born and the happiness that the coming King will bring.

If you want to find out more Jesus and on how to get saved, please see the back of this book under *Other Useful Resources*. I can promise you that once you understand this message, you will get rid of your misery and depression.

For now, I will leave you with some verses from the King James Bible, taken from this website:

https://www.kingjamesbibleonline.org/Bible-Verses-About-Depression/

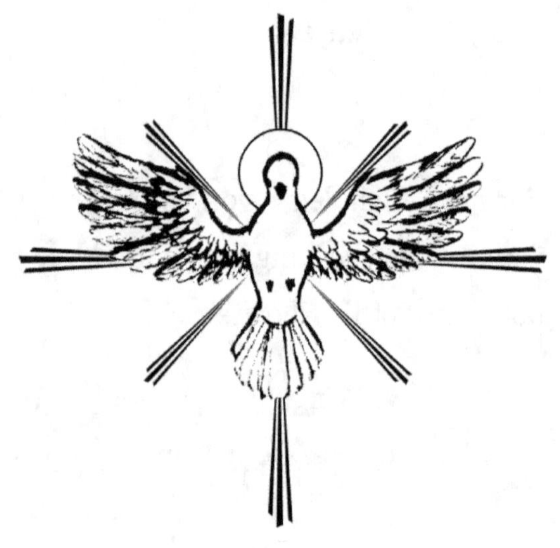

Psalms 34:17-18 – [The righteous] cry, and the LORD heareth, and delivereth them out of all their troubles.

Matthew 11:28 – Come unto me, all [ye] that labour and are heavy laden, and I will give you rest.

1 Peter 5:7 – Casting all your care upon him; for he careth for you.

Isaiah 41:10 – Fear thou not; for I [am] with thee: be not dismayed; for I [am] thy God: I will strengthen thee; yea, I will help thee; yea, I will uphold thee with the right hand of my righteousness.

Jeremiah 29:11 – For I know the thoughts that I think toward you, saith the LORD, thoughts of peace, and not of evil, to give you an expected end.

Proverbs 3:5-6 – Trust in the LORD with all thine heart; and lean not unto thine own understanding.

Psalms 30:5 – For his anger [endureth but] a moment; in his favour [is] life: weeping may endure for a night, but joy [cometh] in the morning.

Psalms 143:7 – 127:8 – Hear me speedily, O LORD: my spirit faileth:

hide not thy face from me, lest I be like unto them that go down into the pit.

Philippians 4:6-7 – Be careful for nothing; but in every thing by prayer and supplication with thanksgiving let your requests be made known unto God.

Psalms 23:4 – Yea, though I walk through the valley of the shadow of death, I will fear no evil: for thou [art] with me; thy rod and thy staff they comfort me.

Romans 12:2 – And be not conformed to this world: but be ye

transformed by the renewing of your
mind, that ye may prove what [is]
that good, and acceptable, and
perfect, will of God.

Proverbs 12:25 – Heaviness in the
heart of man maketh it stoop: but a
good word maketh it glad.

Psalms 9:9 – The LORD also will
be a refuge for the oppressed, a
refuge in times of trouble.

2 Timothy 1:7 – For God hath not
given us the spirit of fear; but of
power, and of love, and of a sound
mind.

Psalms 34:18 – The LORD [is] nigh unto them that are of a broken heart; and saveth such as be of a contrite spirit.

Revelation 21:4 – And God shall wipe away all tears from their eyes; and there shall be no more death, neither sorrow, nor crying, neither shall there be any more pain: for the former things are passed away.

John 10:10 – The thief cometh not, but for to steal, and to kill, and to destroy: I am come that they might have life, and that they might have [it] more abundantly.

(King James Bible)

I highly recommend that you read the gospel of John if you are new to the bible. In the gospel of John, we learn about joy and that it is found in God, through Christ, like a branch that connected to a vine. Christ our vine, our life source, and all we need to do is stay connected to the life source and cared for, and this includes pruning away that which is not beneficial to our growth. In this way, we can grow and flourish in abundance and joy. This inner joy is an everflowing stream that defies all circumstances, predicted by the good news that Jesus was and is God from ancient times, who was born a human, judged by world powers, yet he was perfect and without sin. He bore all our sins, he bore our guilt, sorrow, pain, grief and sickness, atoning our sins bridging the gap between him and us, reconciling us to a relationship with God once again. Jesus shed his blood for us; he conquered death, hell and burial, giving us the gift of hope and eternal life, peace and joy forever more, as it was meant to be in the beginning, in the garden of Eden.

This world is a temporary place, and Jesus is coming back very soon. Make sure you are ready and form a relationship with him today.

We are all sinners Romans 3:23 deserving of death including both physical death and eternal torment in the lake of fire, but you can have eternal life John 15:13. God died for our sins 1 Cor. 15:3, 4, and also Isaiah. 53: 6.

There are four things that you must accept to get this assurance. This free gift must be received by you Romans. 6:23b and Acts 16:29-31.

It is important to know that believing on Christ is not only about acknowledging that the events in the bible happened, but that it is in TRUSTING His substitutionary death, burial, and resurrection for his salvation.

You must trust Christ from your heart. For assurance of being saved read John. 3:36. Confess your sins Rom. 10:11. Shortly, consider baptism, church membership and Christian life.

Thank you for reading this book. I sincerely hope and wish it assists you to get over whatever hurdles you face and to begin living the life you want.

Among the tools presented to you in this book to help you overcome depression, you can take action to adjust and remedy some issues that you may have in your life. You can also seek professional help, but on balance, without sounding too preachy, I do ultimately believe that Jesus Christ is the only true way to real happiness, hope, joy and fulfilment. Please check out the links and *Other Useful Resources* page in the back of this book.

Always remember, there is hope and joy ahead for you whatever circumstance you are going through in life but, choose remedying wisely and consider your path carefully.

Best of luck!

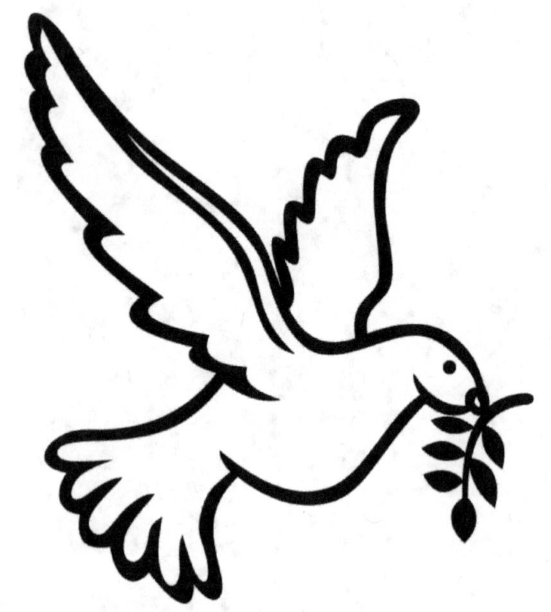

About the Author

Stirling De Cruz-Coleridge published author, philanthropist and entrepreneur. He has written and published several paperbacks, digital books and audiobooks.

He is just a fairly regular guy who left his full-time day job a few years ago and found his voice writing books. The thing about Stirling is that he has experience in many things and enjoys doing various pursuits, often at the same time! Multi-tasking some would call it. He loves to write, enjoys reading, and playing a few instruments plus other fun stuff, while he works on my business.

He is proud of his achievements, like learning to build his website from scratch! He can guarantee you that the books and website articles you will read can impact on your life, in the best possible ways.

Stirling hopes that you get as much value from his books as he intended it to deliver.

Thank you once again for reading this book, and for your patience. Please check out the rest of his books and have a wonderfully productive day, with every success!

If you found this book helpful/useful, please leave an honest review and thanks!

Books by This Author

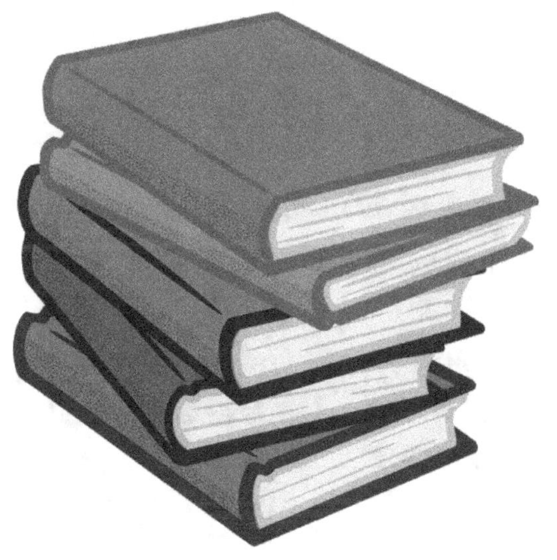

<u>Live Your Life with Success, Good Habits and Love: 45 Highly Effective Habits of Successful People</u>
<u>Authored by Stirling De Cruz-Coleridge</u> (book/*FREE audiobooks when you sign up for Audible 30 Day Trial*).

<u>**Get Back Your Confidence and Learn to Love Yourself After a Relationship Breakup: Self-Love, Personal Transformation, Self-Esteem, Emotional Healing, Self-Improvement & Self-Confidence, Motivation**</u>
<u>Authored by Stirling De Cruz-</u>

<u>Coleridge</u> (book/audible).

<u>**Learning and Memory: How to Use Advanced Strategies & Techniques to Remember More, Learn More, Accelerate Your Brain Power & How to Avoid Memory Deficit in Later Life**</u>
<u>Authored by Stirling De Cruz-</u>

<u>Coleridge</u> (book/audible).

<u>**Personal Transformation and**</u>

<u>**Emotional Healing after a**</u>

<u>**Relationship** *Breakup (Personal*</u>

Transformation, Relationship Breakup,
Emotional Healing, Self Esteem, Self
Confidence, Self Improvement)
(book/audible).

Personal Transformation Habits, Happiness and Success (Success, Live Life, Love).

Powerful, Motivational Success Habits and Personal Transformation: 10 Effective Ways to Create Self Confidence and an Awesome Life (book/audible).

Positive Thinking: Develop Your Emotional Muscles to Achieve Success & Happiness.

Success, Happiness, Power and Money: How to Make Your Life

Awesome in 15 Ways (Personal Transformation, Motivational, Self-Esteem, Happiness Book 2) (book/audible).

Maximise Your Success
Online: Social Media & Digital Marketing for Beginners Tips & Tricks.

Self-Publishing Success

Guide: Step by Step Beginner to Intermediate Guide How to Create and Publish Your E-Book.

Visit Stirling De Cruz Coleridge's website

For training courses, please go to:

https://maximiseyoursuccessonline.com/useful-links/

https://maximiseyoursuccessonline.com/overcome depression

Other Useful Resources

https://www.bbcenglish.org/

https://www.biblestudytools.com/topical-verses/bible-verses-to-comfort-you/

https://www.biblestudytools.com/topical-verses/healing-bible-verses/

https://www.biblestudytools.com/topical-verses/faith-bible-verses/

https://www.biblestudytools.com/topical-verses/bible-verses-for-overcoming-grief/

https://www.biblestudytools.com/topical-verses/worry-and-anxiety-bible-verses/

https://www.biblestudytools.com/topical-verses/bible-verses-about-cancer/

The King James Bible Believing
Church, for those with nowhere else
to go:

https://www.thecloudchurch.org

www.ingramcontent.com/pod-product-compliance
Lightning Source LLC
Chambersburg PA
CBHW071207240726
48654CB00009B/684